Your *Clinics* subscri... ...tter!

You can now access the FULL TEXT of this publication online at no additional cost! Activate your online subscription today and receive...

- Full text of all issues from 2002 to the present
- Photographs, tables, illustrations, and references
- Comprehensive search capabilities
- Links to MEDLINE and Elsevier journals

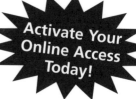

Activate Your Online Access Today!

Plus, you can also sign up for E-alerts of upcoming issues or articles that interest you, and take advantage of exclusive access to bonus features!

To activate your individual online subscription:

1. Visit our website at **www.TheClinics.com**.

2. Click on "Register" at the top of the page, and follow the instructions.

3. To activate your account, you will need your subscriber account number, which you can find on your mailing label (note: the number of digits in your subscriber account number varies from six to ten digits). See the sample below where the subscriber account number has been circled.

This is your subscriber account number

```
************************************************3-DIGIT 001
FEB00   J0167   C7   123456-89   10/00   Q: 1

J.H. DOE, MD
531 MAIN ST
CENTER CITY, NY  10001-001
```

4. That's it! Your online access to the most trusted source for clinical reviews is now available.

theclinics.com

ELSEVIER

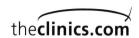

CLINICS IN PODIATRIC MEDICINE AND SURGERY OF NORTH AMERICA

Osteotomies of the
Foot and Ankle

GUEST EDITOR
D. Martin Chaney, DPM, FACFAS

CONSULTING EDITOR
Vincent J. Mandracchia, DPM, MS

April 2005 • Volume 22 • Number 2

SAUNDERS

An Imprint of Elsevier, Inc.
PHILADELPHIA   LONDON   TORONTO   MONTREAL   SYDNEY   TOKYO

W.B. SAUNDERS COMPANY
A Division of Elsevier Inc.

The Curtis Center • Independence Square West • Philadelphia, Pennsylvania 19106

http://www.theclinics.com

CLINICS IN PODIATRIC MEDICINE
AND SURGERY   Volume 22, Number 2
April 2005   ISSN 0891-8422
Editor: Karen Sorensen   ISBN 1-4160-2707-6

The ideas and opinions expressed in *Clinics in Podiatric Medicine and Surgery* do not necessarily reflect those of the Publisher. The Publisher does not assume any responsibility for any injury and/or damage to persons or property arising out of or related to any use of the material contained in this periodical. The reader is advised to check the appropriate medical literature and the product information currently provided by the manufacturer of each drug to be administered to verify the dosage, the method and duration of administration, or contraindications. It is the responsibility of the treating physician or other health care professional, relying on independent experience and knowledge of the patient, to determine drug dosages and the best treatment for the patient. Mention of any product in this issue should not be construed as endorsement by the contributors, editors, or the Publisher of the product or manufacturers' claims.

Reprints. For copies of 100 or more of articles in this publication, please contact the Commercial Reprints Department, Elsevier Inc., 360 Park Avenue South, New York, New York 10010-1710 Tel.: (212) 633-3813, Fax: (212) 462-1935, e-mail: reprints@elsevier.com

Clinics in Podiatric Medicine and Surgery (ISSN 0891-8422) is published quarterly by Elsevier. Corporate and editorial Offices: 170 S Independence Mall W 300 E, Philadelphia, PA 19106–3399. Accounting and circulation offices: 6277 Sea Harbor Drive, Orlando, FL 32887–4800. Periodicals postage paid at Orlando, FL 32862, and additional mailing offices. Subscription prices are $170.00 per year for US individuals, $266.00 per year for US institutions, $85.00 per year for US students and residents, $205.00 per year for Canadian individuals, $322.00 per year for Canadian institutions, $225.00 for international individuals, $322.00 for international institutions and $113.00 per year for Canadian and foreign students/residents. To receive student/resident rate, orders must be accompanied by name of affiliated institution, date of term, and the *signature* of program/residency coordinator on institution letterhead. Orders will be billed at individual rate until proof of status is received. Foreign air speed delivery is included in all *Clinics* subscription prices. All prices are subject to change without notice. POSTMASTER: Send address changes to *Clinics in Podiatric Medicine and Surgery*, W.B. Saunders Company, Periodicals Fulfillment, Orlando, FL 32887-4800. **Customer Service: 1-800-654-2452 (US). From outside of the US, call 1-407-345-1000.**

Clinics in Podiatric Medicine and Surgery is covered in *Index Medicus* and *EMBASE/ Excerpta Medica.*

Printed in the United States of America.

CONSULTING EDITOR

VINCENT J. MANDRACCHIA, DPM, MS, Section Chief, Podiatric Surgery, Department of Surgery, Broadlawns Medical Center; and Clinical Professor, Department of Podiatric Medicine and Surgery, College of Podiatric Medicine and Surgery, Des Moines University–Osteopathic Medicine Center, Des Moines, Iowa

GUEST EDITOR

D. MARTIN CHANEY, DPM, FACFAS, Alamo Family Foot & Ankle Care, San Antonio, Texas

CONTRIBUTORS

BRIAN E. DeYOE, DPM, FACFAS, Podiatric Surgical Associates of North Texas, Baylor University Medical Center, Dallas, Texas

LAWRENCE A. DiDOMENICO, DPM, FACFAS, Director, Youngstown Podiatric Residency Program, Forum Health, Youngstown, Ohio; Adjunct Professor, Ohio College of Podiatric Medicine, Cleveland, Ohio

RYAN P. FRANK, DPM, Podiatric Surgical Residency, Medical Center of Independence, Independence, Missouri

LARRY R. GOSS, DPM, FACFAS, FACFAOM, Director, Parkview/Roxborough/MCP Podiatric Surgical Residency Programs; Clinical Instructor, Temple University School of Podiatric Medicine, Philadelphia, Pennsylvania

THOMAS W. GRONER, DPM, Third-Year Resident, Youngstown Podiatric Residency Program, Forum Health, Youngstown, Ohio

JEFF HETMAN, DPM, Assistant Director, West Houston Medical Center, Harris County Podiatric Surgical Residency Program, Houston, Texas; Private Practice, Houston, Texas

MICHAEL S. LEE, DPM, FACFAS, Central Iowa Orthopaedics, Des Moines, Iowa

KEVIN D. MYER, DPM, West Houston Medical Center, Harris County Podiatric Surgical Residency Program, Houston, Texas

FLOYD PACHECO, DPM, Fourth-Year Resident, Mercy Hospital/Barry University, Miami Shores, Florida

STEPHEN C. ROBINSON, DPM, Residency Director 1995–2002, 2004 to Present; Rotating Podiatric Residency and Podiatric Surgical Residency, Medical Center of Independence, Independence, Missouri

MATTHEW S. ROCKETT, DPM, FACFAS, Bay Area Podiatry Associates, Houston, Texas

THOMAS S. ROUKIS, DPM, Weil Foot and Ankle Institute, Des Plaines, Illinois

GEORGE VITO, DPM, Director, The Atlanta Leg Deformity Correction Center, Macon, Georgia

JEREMY WOOD, DPM, Resident, Presbyterian Medical Center of Greenville, Greenville, Texas

CONTENTS

> This article discusses various forms of distal metatarsal osteotomy
> for the treatment of hallux valgus. The techniques for the various
> osteotomies have evolved over the years to allow the surgeon to
> match a procedure and its modifications to the individual patient's
> deformity, thus optimizing outcomes. Fixation techniques continue
> to evolve, and meticulous surgical technique to prevent complica-
> tions remains a must. Regardless of the osteotomy used, the authors
> believe that adherence to the techniques laid out in current litera-
> ture will provide gratifying results for the surgeon and the patient.

> In this article, the authors describe the indications, contraindica-
> tions, surgical technique and its fixation considerations, postoper-
> ative care, results, and potential complications of the offset V and
> the traditional Z osteotomies. Because of its versatility, inherent
> stability, minimal first metatarsal shortening, good intermetatarsal
> reduction, and ease of rigid internal fixation, shaft osteotomies are
> gaining popularity as procedures for the correction of hallux valgus.
> Strong and stable internal fixation allows for earlier functional
> recovery and primary bone healing. Shaft osteotomies can provide
> predictable and rewarding results for the patient and surgeon for
> the correction of hallux valgus.

Central Metatarsal Head-Neck Osteotomies: Indications and Operative Techniques

Thomas S. Roukis

The author presents the history and indications of various central metatarsal head-neck osteotomies with special emphasis on the radiographic assessment, vascular supply, and regional anatomy. The surgical techniques described include (1) minimal incision osteotomy; (2) Weil metatarsal osteotomy and various modifications; and (3) a novel "telescoping" osteotomy. Ancillary soft-tissue and osseous digital procedures as well as the prevention and management of potential complications are presented in detail.

The Tailor's Bunionette Deformity: A Field Guide to Surgical Correction

Thomas S. Roukis

The author presents a detailed review of the Tailor's bunionette deformity of the fifth metatarsal with special emphasis on radiographic analysis and surgical correction. The surgical techniques discussed include (1) partial metatarsal head ostectomy; (2) metatarsal head resection; (3) minimal incision osteotomy; (4) osteotomies about the metatarsal head-neck, shaft, and base; and (5) ancillary soft tissue procedures. Techniques employed to prevent and correct potential complications are discussed in detail for each osteotomy.

Midfoot Osteotomies for the Cavus Foot

Thomas W. Groner and Lawrence A. DiDomenico

Midfoot osteotomies have long been used for a wide variety of congenital and acquired deformities. Severe pes cavus often necessitates some form of surgical correction, and no single procedure can be used exclusively. Midfoot osteotomies may be combined with adjunctive procedures to form an appropriate strategy for the treatment of these deformities. The authors present an overview of pes cavus, including evaluation and classification of the deformity, as well as associated conditions. Several soft tissue and osseous procedures for correction of the cavus foot are discussed. Special attention is directed at the use of various midfoot osteotomies and their ability to enhance such correction.

The Evans Calcaneal Osteotomy

Brian E. DeYoe and Jeremy Wood

The Evans calcaneal osteotomy is currently the premier procedure for lateral column lengthening of the flexible flatfoot deformity. It has withstood the test of time, proving itself an effective procedure for the correction of pediatric flexible flatfoot. Current understanding of the osteotomy has allowed the Evans calcaneal osteotomy to become a useful tool in the correction of the adult flexible flatfoot as well.

FORTHCOMING ISSUES

RECENT ISSUES

THE CLINICS ARE NOW AVAILABLE ONLINE!

http://www.theclinics.com

ELSEVIER
SAUNDERS

Clin Podiatr Med Surg
22 (2005) ix–x

CLINICS IN
PODIATRIC
MEDICINE AND
SURGERY

Foreword

Osteotomies of the Foot and Ankle

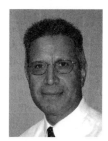

Vincent J. Mandracchia, DPM, MS
Consulting Editor

If you can dodge a wrench, you can dodge a ball.

—Patches O'Houlihan, 2004

My 11-year-old son kept bugging me about taking Tae Kwon Do lessons. Finally, after months of begging and pleading, I told my wife to go ahead and sign him up for classes. About a week later, my wife informed me that we all were registered for Tae Kwon Do. I looked at her and said, "define *all*." Subsequently, I have been involved in the martial arts, with my entire family, for the past 6 months.

We are very fortunate to have instructors who understand the martial arts— not just the forms, blocks, kicks, and punches, but more importantly, the philosophy, the way of life. They spend as much time explaining the role of Tae Kwon Do in every aspect of life as they do the self-defense aspects. This is a great experience for my children and, quite frankly, for me as well. One very important understanding is the concept of yin and yang, the balance in one's life. The yin and yang represent opposites, opposing one another in their actions, and each of these opposites produces the other. According to Chinese philosophy, the production of yin from yang and yang from yin occurs cyclically and constantly, so that no one principle continually dominates the other or determines the other.

0891-8422/05/$ – see front matter © 2005 Elsevier Inc. All rights reserved.
doi:10.1016/j.cpm.2005.01.002
podiatric.theclinics.com

So, this got me to thinking about podiatry. I have been actively involved in the training of students and residents for the past 28 years, and I wonder if I have taught them the application of yin and yang, for I believe that there should be a balance in our professional lives. Have I taught them, through my word and own actions, that podiatric medicine, being a doctor is a way of life, a lifestyle that exudes compassion, understanding, empathy, and humility in our everyday encounters? Have I shown them the balance between family and profession, or is it just about ego, finances, and prestige? Isn't there balance within our own profession, conservative versus surgical care, decision making taking the patient and their lifestyle into account? As I look around me I see tremendous application of this balance in life.

I guess you can teach an old dog new tricks. I know that I will be approaching students and residents differently. I have a better understanding of balance in my life, and as I endeavor to achieve that balance, I will attempt to help the students and residents achieve the same. It is a simple yet profoundly wonderful concept.

Vincent J. Mandracchia, DPM, MS
Broadlawns Medical Center
1801 Hickman Road
Des Moines, IA 50314, USA
E-mail address: vmandracchia@broadlawns.org

ELSEVIER
SAUNDERS

Clin Podiatr Med Surg
22 (2005) xi

CLINICS IN
PODIATRIC
MEDICINE AND
SURGERY

Preface

Osteotomies of the Foot and Ankle

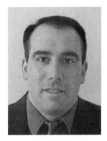

D. Martin Chaney, DPM, FACFAS
Guest Editor

Nowhere in the human body do physicians use osteotomies more often than in foot and ankle surgery. As foot and ankle surgeons, we are required to be proficient in power cutting instrumentation, deformity realignment, and fixation.

In this issue of the *Clinics in Podiatric Medicine and Surgery*, we attempt to cover a wide variety of osteotomy techniques used today in foot and ankle surgery. Our goal is to enhance the reader's understanding of the appropriate indications for the use of these techniques and to share technique "pearls" for direct application. These osteotomies are used to treat a wide variety of foot and ankle pathologies commonly seen today.

It has been my honor to serve as Guest Editor of this issue. I hope you will find this assembly of fine articles enhances your understanding of this powerful surgical technique.

D. Martin Chaney, DPM, FACFAS
Alamo Family Foot & Ankle Care
7424 Broadway
San Antonio, TX 78209, USA
E-mail address: marty.chaney@gmail.com

doi:10.1016/j.cpm.2005.01.001
podiatric.theclinics.com

ELSEVIER
SAUNDERS

Clin Podiatr Med Surg
22 (2005) 143–167

CLINICS IN
PODIATRIC
MEDICINE AND
SURGERY

The Distal Metatarsal Osteotomy for the Treatment of Hallux Valgus

Jeff Hetman, DPM*, Kevin D. Myer, DPM[1]

*West Houston Medical Center, Harris County Podiatric Surgical Residency Program,
11301 Richmond Avenue, Suite K-105, Houston, TX 77082, USA*

For over 100 years there have been many procedures described for the correction of hallux abductovalgus deformities, ranging from the simple "bumpectomy" to complex basalar osteotomies and fusions. Each procedure was developed, and in many cases modified over time, to either address the specific or "dominant" part of the deformity or to create a procedure that was superior in achieving correction while minimizing potential complications and increasing the likelihood of a good outcome. Of these many procedures, the ones that achieve correction at the distal aspect of the metatarsal have historically been, and have remained, the most popular. These procedures have retained their popularity for many reasons, including postoperative weight-bearing status, low risk of postoperative complications, ability to address deformities in more than one plane and, in some cases, technical ease.

All distal metatarsal osteotomy (DMO) procedures are typically performed for intermetatarsal angles of 15 degrees or less, although there is literature that suggests the success of these osteotomies with greater intermetatarsal (IM) angles. Controversy still remains regarding the potential for avascular necrosis of the head of the metatarsal following a DMO as there is literature that supports both the tendency of and the tendency against this complication occurring. The efficacy of types and techniques of fixation of DMOs is also coming to the forefront of the literature.

---

* Corresponding author.
E-mail address: jhetman@sbcglobal.net (J. Hetman).
[1] Article submitted during second year of residency.

0891-8422/05/$ – see front matter © 2005 Elsevier Inc. All rights reserved.
doi:10.1016/j.cpm.2004.11.001   *podiatric.theclinics.com*

Historical perspective

Hohmann

Hohmann [1] is often mistakenly credited with describing the first meta-tarsal osteotomy for the correction of HAV. The Hohmann bunionectomy was first described in 1921, and published in 1923, as a through-and-through transverse/oblique osteotomy performed at the neck of the metatarsal. The osteotomy is orientated distal-medial to proximal-lateral, and a medial wedge of bone is generally resected. This osteotomy enables the surgeon to achieve triplane correction as it is able to correct for an increased IM angle and an increased proximal articular set angle (PASA) as well as allow for plantar-flexion of the capital fragment. Because of its location at the neck of the metatarsal, the sesamoid apparatus is avoided, which minimizes the chance of developing sesamoid arthritis. The main drawbacks to this procedure are lack of fixation and failure to resect the medial eminence. There is also in-creased recurrence of the HAV deformity reported when performing the Hohmann osteotomy [1a].

Modifications of the Hohmann osteotomy center on the use of internal fixation. In 1984, Warrick and Edelman studied modifications, including resection of the medial eminence of the first metatarsal head and changing the direction of the wedge resection from a transverse to an oblique orientation [2]. They believed that this change of orientation allows for proper screw fixation. This modification was deemed technically difficult to perform because the two osteotomies required to remove a trapezoid wedge violate the medial and lateral cortices of the first metatarsal, which decreases the stability of the first metatarsal. They performed their modified Hohmann bunionectomy on a total of 15 feet and 11 patients. The average preoperative intermetatarsal angle was 12.5 degrees, which was decreased to 7.7 degrees. There was one osteotomy that resulted in a mildly dorsiflexed first metatarsal. They discussed how greater intermetatarsal angle reduction was possible by increasing the obliquity of the osteotomy, but this occurred at the cost of increased shortening of the metatarsal. The width of the first metatarsal shaft was also a limiting factor when determining the amount of correction available, as the surgeon should maintain 33% to 50% of bone contact. The size of the trapezoidal wedge resected from the surgical neck of the metatarsal determines the amount of PASA correction. In their discussion, they pointed out that the most detri-mental complication encountered was the inherent shortening that occurred, on average, of 4.1 mm [2]. They blamed this shortening on the amount of bone resected and the amount of lateral transposition of the capital fragment on an oblique plane. This increasing transposition causes deviation from the strict A-O principles regarding the length of the fracture/osteotomy site in relationship to the shaft diameter. This limits the application of this procedure to the mild to moderate hallux valgus deformity [3–5].

Peabody

In 1931, Peabody reported an osteotomy similar to that of Reverdin, with some improvements [6]. Peabody oriented the osteotomy in the anatomical neck, as did Hohmann, thus avoiding the sesamoid apparatus. He removed a medially based wedge for angular correction and maintained the lateral cortex to prevent horizontal shifting of the capital fragment. But Peabody also resected the medial eminence of the first metatarsal head and employed fixation through the use of heavy chromic suture through drill holes.

The disadvantages of the Peabody osteotomy were that it did not address an increased intermetatarsal angle and did not allow for sagittal plane correction [4].

Mitchell

In 1945, Hawkins et al [7] first described a biplane, double step-off osteotomy, which they claimed was simple, technically. Indications for this osteotomy include valgus deformity of the hallux, exostosis formation, painful metatarso-phalangeal articulation, and the presence of metatarsus primus varus. The original procedure described a double-osteotomy, which resulted in removal of an interposing fragment that was not to exceed one eighth of an inch while maintaining a lateral bony strut whose width ranged from one half to five sixths of the width of the metatarsal, depending on the foot type and amount of correction desired. The proximal osteotomy was then completed, resulting in a lateral bony spicule that was maintained on the capital fragment, and the capital fragment was laterally displaced and impacted so that the lateral spicule was secure against the lateral shaft of the metatarsal. Fixation was created with heavy chromic suture and hallux repositioning was achieved with medial capsulor-rhaphy and postoperative splinting. This technique allowed for reduction of the IM angle and reduction of any sagittal plane deformity [8–11].

Several potential complications of this osteotomy are described in the literature. The technical demand of this procedure is great because of the removal of a rectangular wedge while retaining a lateral cortical spike. Wedge removal also results in shortening, which can lead to lesser metatarsalgia. Risks of increased angulation and displacement are also possible because of the osteotomy's inherent instability. Some authors also suggest increased risk of postoperative restriction of motion and deformity recurrence. Although most patients are allowed to bear weight immediately following most distal metatarsal osteotomies, patients undergoing this procedure must maintain non–weight bearing for a short period of time [4].

Several modifications of the Mitchell osteotomy have been developed to simplify it. The Wu modification included an oblique orientation that allowed for plantar transposition to compensate for the metatarsal shortening [11]. Weiner et al [11a,11b] also addressed the shortening component of the Mitchell by describing a trapezoidal wedge in which the medial border was shorter than the lateral. Roux described the opposite, with the lateral border being shorter than the medial. He also claimed that this allowed for further correction of an increased PASA [8–12].

Wilson

The Wilson osteotomy was described in 1963 as a through-and-through osteotomy orientated 45 degrees to the transverse plane, beginning at the proximal aspect of the medial eminence and running in a distal-medial to proximal-lateral direction [13]. This osteotomy addressed deformities in the IM angle and the PASA. Through the years following his description of this procedure, several complications were reported in the literature. Shortening was a significant problem because of the orientation of the osteotomy. Inherent instability led to complications of dorsiflexion and malposition of the capital fragment. These two complications combined to cause an increased incidence in lesser metatarsalgia. Other complications included increased recurrence, loss of correction, malunion, and delayed and nonunion [4,14–16].

To reduce some of these complications, several modifications of the Wilson osteotomy were created. Helal et al modified the original Wilson osteotomy by orientating the osteotomy 45 degrees to the sagital plane from a dorsal-distal to plantar-proximal direction, which allowed for the prevention of dorsiflexion seen with the original Wilson osteotomy [14a]. To compensate for any shortening that might occur, plantarflexion of the capital fragment can be performed [14–16].

Klareskov et al modified Wilson's osteotomy by plantarflexing the capital fragment as it was displaced laterally, which accommodated for the excessive shortening commonly encountered [14b]. This reduced the weight-bearing reactive forces on the lateral metatarsal heads. However, it is reported that even with this modification, dorsal angulation of the capital fragment is common [4].

Another modification by Grace et al [15] reinforced the medial capsule by suturing a medial flap of capsule under tension to the periosteum or through a drill hole in the metatarsal shaft. Even with this modification, however, the authors noted up to 10 patients who experienced a loss of position after the metatarsal head had been displaced laterally [15].

Allen et al were the first to use internal fixation [15a]. They used a cancellous screw to fixate a medially based wedge, which allowed for simultaneous correction of a laterally deviated cartilaginous surface and increased IM angle [14].

Geldwert et al [14] observed 115 feet that underwent a Wilson osteotomy for the correction of hallux abductovalgus using various forms of fixation, such as cortical and cancellous screws as well as crossing Kirschner wires. In this study, the authors concluded that 80% of these procedures performed ended with either excellent or good results with only one complication, that being a hallux varus [14].

As suggested by White [16] in his article "Variations of the Wilson Bunionectomy," although he performs this osteotomy on the active patient, he prefers to reserve it for the less functional foot. In a review of his patients, he notes that three of four surgeries resulted in limited motion secondary to iatrogenic primus elevatus from the osteotomy being performed too close to the midshaft of the metatarsal [16].

In 1988, Grace et al [15] performed a retrospective study comparing the results of 31 Wilson and 31 Hohmann osteotomies of the first metatarsal for the correction of hallux valgus. Most patients reported higher than 50% satisfaction after both operations, although few patients reported that they were totally satisfied with their results. The Hohmann osteotomy produced more variability with patient satisfaction. Two thirds of the patients were completely pain-free at follow-up with only a small number of feet remaining painful after both osteotomies. The average improvement in the hallux valgus and first intermetatarsal angles were similar for both osteotomies, and the amount of shortening was similar (Wilson 6.3%; Hohmann 6.4%). Degenerative changes about the first MPJ occurred more frequently following the Hohmann procedure versus the Wilson despite that fewer feet in the former group showed preexisting changes. Pedobarographic studies demonstrated that most feet in both osteotomy groups produced isolated peak loading under a single lateral metatarsal head, most often the second metatarsal. Nine feet in the Wilson group showed maximum loading under the lateral three metatarsal heads compared with only two feet in the Hohmann group. There were no serious complications. Seven patients were dissatisfied in the Wilson group and seven in the Hohmann group. Dissatisfaction in the Wilson group was attributed to recurrence in deformity and stiffness in the joint, pain in the first MPJ, pain within the second digit, recurrence with metatarsalgia, and one functionless hallux with painful callosities. In the Hohmann group, dissatisfaction was due to metatarsalgia, recurrence of the deformity with and without pain, and joint stiffness [15].

Reverdin

Reverdin [17] described the first osteotomy for the correction of HAV in 1881. This procedure consisted of a medially based wedge osteotomy in the frontal plane, which maintained an intact lateral hinge. The osteotomy is from dorsal to plantar proximal to the articular surface of the metatarsal but distal to the sesamoid apparatus. The original goals of this procedure were to correct the PASA and achieve some reduction of the IM angle, the latter incidental to the reverse buckling that occurs with closure of the osteotomy with the intact lateral hinge. Reverdin [17] believed that up to 3.5 degrees of correction could be achieved with this reverse buckling phenomenon.

The original Reverdin osteotomy was associated with difficult fixation because of the transverse orientation of the osteotomy and potential sesamoid trauma. Therefore, several modifications evolved to address these shortcomings when performing the procedure. The Green modification used an oblique plantar arm to avoid disruption of the sesamoid articulation. Green [18] maintained the lateral hinge and therefore his modification did not address the intermetatarsal angle or sagittal plane deformities.

The Laird modification, first described in 1977, is essentially identical to the Reverdin-Green modification, but the osteotomy is continued through the lateral cortex. This modification not only allowed for correction of PASA but also for reduction of an increased IM angle. In 1988, Laird modified the osteotomy further by resecting a medially based wedge of bone from the plantar shaft of the metatarsal to reduce valgus rotation of the great toe. He also stated that metatarsal length could be preserved if the proximal aspect of the dorsal osteotomy was oriented more perpendicular to the metatarsal shaft than to the frontal body plane [18].

Another interesting modification was introduced by Zyzda and Hineser [19] in 1989, which used bone graft to alleviate potential shortening and a grafting technique to correct sagital plane deformity. If the PASA was large or the metatarsal short, they proposed rotating the resected dorsal wedge of bone 180° and reinserting it into the dorsal osteotomy site with the base oriented laterally as an autogenous bone graft. To avoid overcorrection, they stated that the width of the base should be one half of the necessary width to correct the PASA deformity. They also stated that sagittal plane and rotational deformities could be addressed with grafting techniques as opposed to the techniques described by Todd and Laird [18]. For correction of valgus deformity, they propose inserting the resected wedge into the plantar osteotomy with the base of the wedge lateral. They believe this technique prevents excessive bone resection and therefore excessive correction. They also advocated insertion of a rectangular graft into the plantar osteotomy site for plantarflexion of the metatarsal head, stating that this was more effective than the Todd modification in that it overcame the limitations of the Todd modification and avoided possible overcorrection.

The Reverdin [17] procedure remains a useful alternative today, though it seems to be rarely used as a stand-alone procedure. The authors speculate that this is due to the osteotomy's inherent lack of fixation alternatives, as most literature describes K-wires as the fixation of choice. It is, however, often added as an adjunct procedure to basalar osteotomies or arthrodesis to correct a large PASA. The authors will occasionally add this procedure to a Lapidus procedure, as described by Lombardi et al [20], when soft tissue correction of the valgus deformity is insufficient or the PASA is particularly large. Though significant shortening of the first metatarsal occurs with this combined procedure, the authors, like Lombardi, have found no incidence of lesser metatarsalgia complaints, which can be attributed to adequate plantarflexion of the metatarsal at the arthrodesis site.

Reverdin-Laird tips

When performing a Reverdin-Laird-type osteotomy, create the plantar osteotomy first and detach the saw blade from the saw and leave it in the plantar osteotomy site. This will serve as a rigid "stop" to prevent the accidental resection of the plantar shelf while creating the dorsal osteotomies (Fig. 1). When creating the dorsal wedge osteotomy, always resect far less of a wedge than is originally estimated. It may be beneficial to draw the wedge on the dorsal aspect

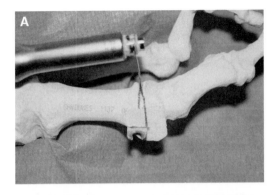

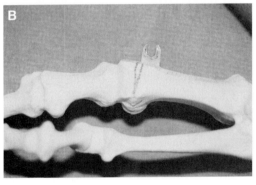

Fig. 1. (*A*) AP view of plantar cut with saw blade for stop. (*B*) Lateral view, creating dorsal cuts with saw blade for stop.

of the metatarsal and then stay within those boundaries, taking into account the width of the saw blade. Creating the dorsal wedge apex short of the lateral cortex will result in a true wedge formation and not a trapezoidal configuration, which would minimize the amount of correction achieved (Fig. 2).

Austin

In 1962, Austin first proposed and performed a horizontally directed "V" displacement osteotomy for correction of hallux valgus [21]. In 1981, Austin and Leventen [21] published their review of over 1200 patients in which the chevron osteotomy was used; their patient age range was 8 years to 76 years. They believed that bunion correction should restore the alignment of the first metatarsophalangeal joint, correct the hallux valgus and the metatarsus primus varus deformity. Their goal was to develop a procedure that addressed these three key points while maintaining osteotomy stability and allowing for early ambulation.

In a 1981 article, Austin and Leventen [21] stated that indications for the chevron procedure include symptomatic patients with mild to moderate hallux

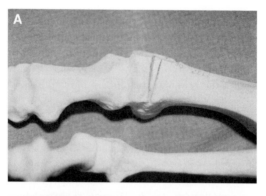

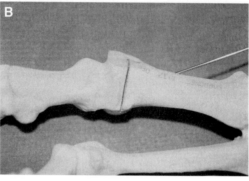

Fig. 2. (*A*) Dorsal view of incomplete dorsal wedge cuts. (*B*) Reduced osteotomy following wedge resection.

valgus and primus varus deformities. Over the years, this has been interpreted as an abducted hallux with the medial or dorsomedial prominence of the first metatarsal head, range of motion of the first metatarsophalangeal joint is pain-free and without crepitus, no significant valgus rotation of the hallux is present, and no evidence of tract-bound phenomenon. Radiographic indications included hallux valgus angle of less than 15 degrees, normal distal articular set angle (DASA) and normal PASA, first IM angle less than 15 degrees, absence of degenerative joint disease, and absence of cystic changes throughout the first metatarsal head. Austin and Leventen [21] were never this specific in their original article with regard to these radiographic and clinical indications. However, these indications have remained the standard and unchanged throughout the years, although more indications have surfaced as modifications for the original procedure have been developed.

Austin and Leventen [21] were not the first publish their findings with the chevron bunionectomy. That distinction belongs to Corless in 1976 [22] followed by Johnson et al in 1979 [23]. Both described the chevron osteotomy as a modification to the Mitchell osteotomy that was technically easier to perform and facilitated better results. Johnson et al [23] found that on 26 feet, follow-up evaluation disclosed good pain relief, cosmetic correction, and patient satisfaction. These authors were also the first to describe the potential for fixation of this osteotomy, relating the use of bone peg across the osteotomy site when necessary. Of note, Austin and Leventen [21] were not referenced.

Many studies relate to the efficacy of the chevron bunionectomy, and a few are reviewed here. Velkes et al [24] assessed chevron osteotomies that were an average of 4 years and 7 months postoperative, revealing that more than 90% of the patients were satisfied with their results. They related complications of intraoperative intraarticular fracture of the metatarsal head in five feet, recurrence in three feet, and tilt of the distal fragment in two feet. They concluded, however, that the chevron osteotomy provides a good and lasting result provided the procedure is performed on patients presenting symptomatic hallux valgus with a first intermetatarsal angle between 10° and 18°.

Hetherington et al [25], in conjunction with Steinbock from Orthapadisches Spital in Vienna, Austria, performed a retrospective study of 180 feet that underwent the chevron procedure performed over a 3-year period. The patient population was subdivided into four groups based on whether fixation or capsular reefing was performed during the procedure. They concluded that the chevron procedure would maintain correction and patient satisfaction long term. They also noted no discrepancy between fixated and unfixated osteotomies with regard to long-term clinical radiographs. They did note that capsular reefing provided no benefit with regards to long-term results, but rather an increase in joint stiffness with the capsular reefing group.

Bar-David et al [26] performed a retrospective analysis comparing the distal chevron osteotomy to basilar osteotomies with the first IM angle of 13° to 16°. Their study included 95 osteotomies on 83 patients over a 3-year period with only 33 patients presenting for long-term assessment. Their follow-up study included physical examination, radiographic examination, and subjective questionnaire. They concluded that the chevron osteotomy was preferred in patients presenting a first IM angle of 13° to 16° and a hallux abductus angle of 30° or less.

Steinstra et al [27] in 2002 suggested that the chevron is not limited to the previously accepted standards in that a large lateral displacement of the capital fragment, 40° or greater, is possible with good results. They performed this procedure on 38 feet, 36 relating no limitation of activities, 25 relating no pain, and only 6 requiring a comfort shoe with inserts. There was only one incidence of capital fragment dislocation, 1 day postoperative, which was immediately repaired and went on to heal unremarkably. Fixation options become an issue as the lateral move becomes larger, with K-wires becoming the most viable option. Steinstra et al [27] readily admit that more study is required but feel that the previously accepted parameters for the chevron osteotomy can be expanded.

Chevron tips

The authors have little to offer with regard to major changes in the basic technique of the chevron osteotomy and no need reinvent a procedure that is considered sound. There are, however, some intraoperative technique suggestions

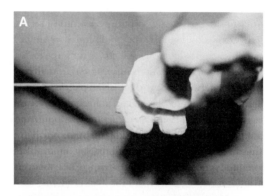

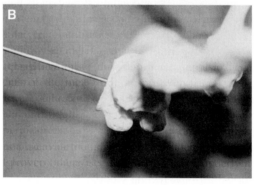

Fig. 3. (*A*) Saw bones depiction of guide wire orientation to stay "on plane." (*B*) Saw bones depiction of guide wire orientation to plantarflex capital fragment.

that can be offered that may make the surgeon's experience with the procedure more precise and more pleasant.

The use of a guide wire to create the osteotomy is an effective method to ensure the surgeon is exact in placement, direction, and congruity of the osteotomy (Fig. 3). An apical axis guide is not necessary to create a uniform bone cut ,and the authors find the axis guide cumbersome as it must be removed to complete the osteotomy at the apex, which could alter the orientation of part of the osteotomy. By keeping the saw blade parallel to wire throughout the cut from medial to lateral, the surgeon can make the osteotomy from apex to cortex in one smooth motion. It is the authors' impression that creating the dorsal or plantar osteotomy in one pass rather than two will also help to minimize the trauma to the bone (Fig. 4). As a side note, the authors' personal preference is to never lavage the osteotomy site during the cuts. If bone burning or smoke occurs while cutting, the procedure should be stopped and the bone allowed to cool. Lavage can be performed at this time but thorough suction of the site should be preformed before resumption of the osteotomy.

If a normal metatarsal parabola is present, the guide wire is oriented from the medial first metatarsal head toward the fourth metatarsal head (Fig 5). This can

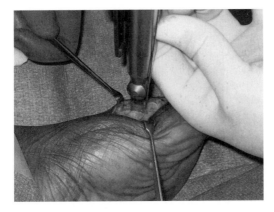

Fig. 4. Using wire as a guide.

be adapted per preoperative assessment of the parabola and adjusted as needed. The guide wire can also assist in lengthening or shortening the metatarsal if necessary. Though the amount of lengthening/shortening that can be achieved is limited, in most cases of mild to moderate HAV the amount needed is usually within the scope of the procedure. The authors also routinely orient the guide wire somewhat plantarflexed (Fig. 6). It has been the authors' experience that it is better to err in a plantarfexory direction rather than attempting to keep the osteotomy in the same plane equal to the preoperative orientation of the forefoot. Preoperative radiographic assessment and intraoperative forefoot loading can give the surgeon a glimpse of the foot position but can in no way mimic the interaction of the foot with the ground during ambulation. Attempting to keep the same sagital plane position of the capital fragment may result in an actual, and inadvertent, dorsiflexion of the head. Mild plantarflexion of the capital fragment avoids this scenario.

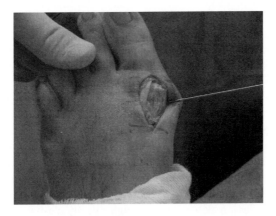

Fig. 5. Guide wire oriented at fourth metatarsal head.

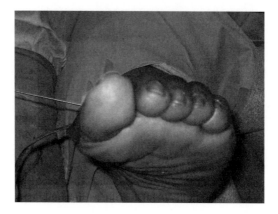

Fig. 6. Plantarflexing guide wire.

The use of a single 0.045-inch K-wire as an osteotomy guide can be extremely beneficial to the experienced surgeon or new practitioner. The authors believe that this 30-second additional step will produce more consistent cuts and predictable position postreduction.

The authors prefer to keep the osteotomy angle at 60° and further recommend creating the plantar portion of the osteotomy initially. This ensures that the osteotomy will avoid the sesamoid apparatus. The authors have found that in keeping the 60° angle there is more than adequate dorsal cortex of the capital fragment to achieve almost any type of rigid internal fixation. Preferred fixation techniques will be reviewed later.

Modifications of the Austin/Chevron osteotomy

Since its inception, and despite predictable and reproducible results of the original described procedure, there been many suggested modifications of the chevron osteotomy. These modifications were developed to increase indications for the procedure with regard to severity of the deformity, to address specific parts of the deformity, to accommodate different types of fixation and to apply to procedure to different pathological situations, such as hallux limitus.

Bicorrectional chevron

It is commonly believed that the chevron, or Austin bunionectomy, was originally described as a transpositional, unicorrectional procedure allowing for reduction of the IM angle while concomitantly allowing for restoration of the congruency of the first metatarsophalangeal joint. However, Austin and Leventen [21] alluded to redirecting the articular surface of the metatarsal head from a valgus to a slight varus position as well as potential correction of angulation, rotation, or dorsiflexion deformities through alteration of the angles of the V osteotomy, if necessary. Although no specific modifications were elaborated upon, the authors believe that this is the first indication that this osteotomy could be used for correction in more than one plane.

Gerbert et al [28] described a transpositional and angulational osteotomy that addressed not only an increased first IM angle but also an abnormal PASA. They described a classic chevron osteotomy from medial to lateral with the addition of the resection of a predetermined wedge of bone from the distal osteotomy site that was angulated to converge at the initial osteotomy laterally. They suggested the initial osteotomy be performed at 80% of the width of the metatarsal, the wedge of bone removed, and then the initial osteotomy completed. Removal of this medially based wedge of bone would facilitate adduction of the capital fragment and thus reduce the PASA. Though long-term results of this modification at the time of publication of this article were not yet available, the short-term results in their patient population were deemed excellent.

Nery et al [29] described a biplanar Chevron osteotomy for the correction of an increased first intermetatarsal angle as well as an increased distal metatarsal articular angle (DMAA). DMAA is the orthopedic equivalent to PASA. This procedure is also described as a chevron osteotomy that includes resection of a dorsal medial wedge of bone from the shaft to reduce the DMAA (PASA). With 61 patients and 104 feet in a 2-year follow-up study, he reported 90% satisfaction rate with no complications, such as AVN, infections, and transfer lesions. Three patients expressed discomfort with prominent fixation and three expressed dissatisfaction with undercorrection, though they were without discomfort. Though this study shows that concomitant correction of a high intermetatarsal angle and increased DMAA (PASA) remains a viable option, correction occurs in only one body plane.

The authors readily use this chevron modification when indicated, adhering to Gerbert's principle and aim for the apex to be short of the lateral cortex, thus creating a true wedge instead of a trapezoidal piece for maximum correction with the least amount of bone resection (Fig. 7).

Youngswick

Youngswick [30] described a different type of modification in 1982 for the treatment of pain in the first metatarsophalangeal joint that clinically presented with decreased motion of the joint and radiographic signs, including metatarsus primus elevatus with evidence of osseous limitation. The original procedure described the creation of the classic chevron osteotomy with a second osteotomy created on the metatarsal shaft parallel to the original dorsal osteotomy, allowing a predetermined portion of bone to be removed. Impaction of the capital fragment on the metatarsal shaft following removal of this portion of bone resulted in plantarflexion of the metatarsal head, thus creating a reduction of the metatarsus primus elevatus. Youngswick [30] maintained the 60° horizontal V osteotomy as described by Austin [21]. This modification can be combined with the lateral displacement of the classic chevron osteotomy, which would then create a true biplanar correction.

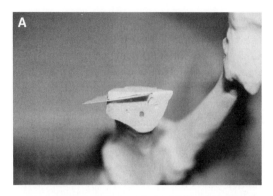

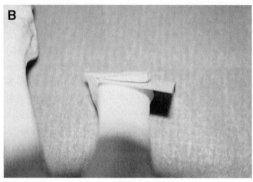

Fig. 7. (*A*) Cross-sectional depiction of creating wedge for bicorrectional chevron. (*B*) Posterior depiction of creating wedge for bicorrectional chevron.

In 2001 Gerbert et al [31] took a more in-depth look at plantar arm orientation and total angle of the Youngswick modification of the chevron osteotomy in relation to a reference line parallel to the ground, the reference line intersecting the apex of the osteotomy. Their study showed that the relationship of the plantar wing angles to the reference line would dictate the amount of shortening or plantarflexion achieved and that dorsal wing orientation had no effect. They felt that for maximum plantarflexion the plantar arm orientation should be 75° to the reference line. They did state, however, that a greater than 60° plantar wing orientation might compromise the stability of the osteotomy and encroach on the sesamoid apparatus. They further speculated that a 30° plantar wing orientation may be ideal for achieving plantar displacement and retaining the stability of the chevron osteotomy.

Tips

The authors deviate from their aforementioned preference and create both dorsal cuts before the plantar cut. Creating the second dorsal cut proximal and parallel to the initial cut before the plantar cut provides a more stable environment. Once both cuts are complete, the surgeon need simply to "connect the dots" while creating the plantar cut and the wedge resection completed without having to try to stabilize an unstable metatarsal shaft (Fig. 8).

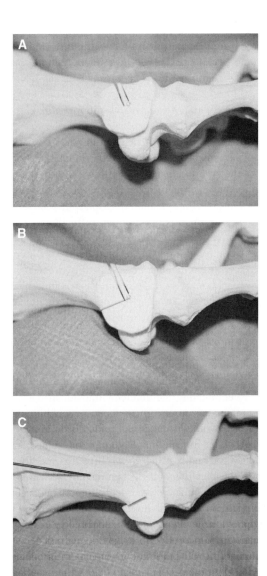

Fig. 8. (*A*) Creating two dorsal cuts for Youngswick modification. (*B*) "Connecting the dots" of the two dorsal cuts. (*C*) Reduced osteotomy, capital fragment plantarflexed.

The authors believe that Gerbert et al's [28] findings are accurate. Another way to look at it is, when creating a Youngswick modification you are creating a new osteotomy apex plantar to the original apex. The vertical distance between the apices will determine the amount of plantarflexion that occurs, if bone resection is constant. The plantar arm angle is determined only by a line drawn between the two apices and its relation to the reference line. An important point is that the plantar apex can *never* be distal to the dorsal apex. Therefore, drawing the plantar wing of the osteotomy and then choosing the apical points on that line before creating the osteotomy will assist the surgeon in avoiding a problem such as invading the sesamoid apparatus or losing structural integrity.

Kalish

In 1983, Kalish first proposed, and then published in 1989 [32], a modification to the standard Austin bunionectomy achieved by closure of the osteotomy angle from 60° to 55°, thus creating a long dorsal wing that facilitated rigid internal fixation. The modification was created to address perceived shortcomings of the standard Austin procedure, including displacement and malposition of the capital fragment, delayed union and nonunion, difficulties with K-wire fixation, and limited postoperative first MPJ range of motion. It also allowed for greater lateral displacement of the capital fragment, thus allowing for correction of larger deformities. However, he readily admitted that this procedure did not address and is not used for reduction of a PASA deformity. His initial study of 264 osteotomies revealed no nonunions or delayed unions [32]. Related complications included hallux varus deformity in 8 of 264 patients, which was attributed to adductor tendon transfer or aggressive medial capsulorrhaphy. In follow-up study in 1994, Kalish [33] examined 265 feet that underwent his modification of the Austin bunionectomy. The procedure performed for this study did not routinely include adductor tendon transfer unless the preoperative IM angle was 15° to 18°. By eliminating the adductor transfer in the patient group with preoperative IM angle of 15° or less, he noted a decrease in postoperative varus deformity. He also believed that the study validated his earlier theory that two-screw fixation is superior because it more evenly distributes compression forces across the osteotomy site and resists rotation of the capital fragment.

In 1992, Downey [34] discussed the many potential pitfalls of the Kalish modification. He stated that this osteotomy required greater technical expertise than a traditional chevron osteotomy and therefore possessed a greater chance of postoperative complications due to technical failure. His conclusion was that most postoperative problems occurred due to a loss of rigid internal fixation but also that the surgeon who paid meticulous attention to the problem areas would achieve gratifying results. There is an interesting technical pearl contained within the body of the article that the authors incorporate into every DMO, that being to create the proximal "free end" of the osteotomy first and work the osteotomy distally toward the apex. By identifying and creating the cortical exit points first, the authors believe that the surgeon will avoid unnecessary dissection and potential soft tissue trauma.

Vogler

The Vogler [5] modification is an osteotomy that combines the concepts of Austin [21], Reverdin [17], and Ludloff [35a]. It is referred to as the "offset V" osteotomy and is truly a shaft osteotomy. It will therefore not be discussed at length in this article.

The authors have incorporated one principle of the offset V into intraoperative decision making with regard to apex placement for a traditional chevron osteotomy. The technique was related to the senior author by Samuel S. Mendicino, DPM, in a personal communication in 1993. When a metatarsal head is more trumpet-shaped than round when viewed laterally, orienting the apex in the traditional fashion may, in some cases, put the osteotomy apex too distal, resulting in a greater chance of fracture of the metatarsal head. In these cir-

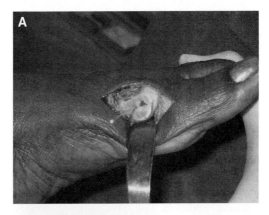

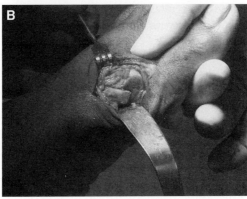

Fig. 9. (*A*) Trumpet-shaped head, note the K-wire is proximally offset. (*B*) Offset chevron postlateral shift of capital fragment.

cumstances, offsetting the osteotomy apex proximally in the fashion described by Vogler eliminates the chance of head fracture and keeps the osteotomy entirely in metaphyseal bone (Fig. 9).

Fixation

The literature abounds in studies for the efficacy of internal fixation, many touting certain types of fixation as superior. Though Austin and Leventen's [21] original description provided for no fixation of the osteotomy, believing that the osteotomy was inherently stable, this thinking is not standard today. It is now readily accepted that fixation of any DMO is necessary for maximum outcome. The best type of fixation, be it the type of fixater, orientation of the fixater, or the proper combination of fixaters, is now coming to the forefront of the literature.

Studies reporting on types of fixation ranging from use of K-wires to soft tissue anchors to the myriad of screw fixaters as well as absorbable options available to today's surgeon are too vast to review here. Many of these publications are simply retrospective studies of a particular physician's experience with a particular style of fixation that has been efficacious for that physician. The authors appreciate this information as there can never be too many options when it comes to fixation of an osteotomy. After all, the goal of fixation is to maintain correction/position while optimizing healing, which in turn provides the surgeon with a good result. An important factor in this mix, however, is the patient. Despite the best efforts of the surgeon, strict instructions, and postoperative restrictions, a patient will occasionally, and inadvertently in most cases, stress an osteotomy site beyond its limitations. For this reason, the authors find the recent research that attempts to identify the strongest type and style of fixation most pertinent today.

Over the past decade, studies by Fox, Shereff, Landsman, Buckenberger, and Chang have compared and contrasted various fixaters with various osteotomies [36a–36e]. In 2003, three independent studies compared fixation strength of the

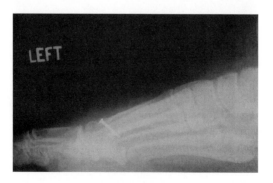

Fig. 10. Chevron fixated with 2.0 screw and absorbable pin.

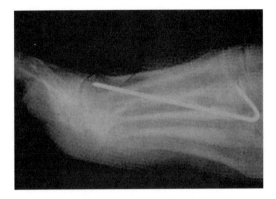

Fig. 11. Chevron fixated with Single K-wire.

offset V osteotomy. Khuri et al [35] looked at load to failure in saw bones where and offset V was fixated with either two 2.0-mm screws, two 2.7-mm screws, two 3.5-mm screws, or one 2.7-mm screw with a single 0.045-inch K-wire. They found no statistical difference in the maximum load sustained between test groups. Dalton et al [36] looked at screw versus K-wire fixation of the offset V in foam and cadaveric specimens, comparing not only the type of fixater but the orientation of the fixater. An interesting part of this study is the addition of a tension band to the cadaveric specimens to attempt to recreate the effects of capsular and ligamentous structures and the stability they provide. They found that the tension band group showed a significantly higher peak load and stiffness.

Jacobson et al [37] studied saw bones load to failure of the offset V fixated with either two 2.0-mm screws, two 2.7-mm screws, one of each screw, or one 2.7-mm screw with a 0.062-inch K-wire, all of the fixation oriented dorsal to plantar parallel to the osteotomy. They found the most stable construct to be the 2.7-mm screw and K-wire.

The authors currently prefer a single 2.0-mm screw from dorsal distal to proximal plantar augmented with a single absorbable pin in the same fashion, oblique to the screw (Fig. 10). The senior author has used many types of fixation,

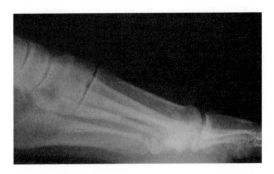

Fig. 12. Chevron fixated with absorbable pins.

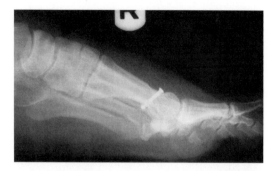

Fig. 13. Chevron fixated with self-locking osteotomy anchor.

including percutaneous K-wires (Fig. 11), absorbable fixation alone (Fig. 12), single screws, two screws, self-locking osteotomy anchors (Fig. 13), and others, with varying results. Though it is the authors' opinion that some type of compression across the osteotomy site is mandatory, and that two-point fixation is becoming the standard, it will be fascinating to see what the future holds with regard to what is the strongest construct for optimum fixation, healing, and avoidance of complication.

Complications and avascular necrosis

The potential for postoperative complications exists with any procedure, and described complications for distal metatarsal osteotomies run the gamut, including malunion, delayed or nonunion, joint stiffness, recurrence, painful hardware if fixation is used, transfer metatarsalgia, osteomyelitis, degenerative joint disease, hallux varus, soft tissue infection, and avascular necrosis. Though all of these complications have been covered in the literature, avascular necrosis (AVN) presents, if not controversy, at least a lively range of opinions as to the occurrence rate, etiology, and prevention.

AVN is defined as death of tissue due to disruption of blood supply, which can ultimately lead to joint collapse. There are many cited causes of AVN when a DMO is performed. These include excessive soft tissue stripping, osteotomy with concomitant lateral release, burning of bone with power instrumentation, fixation (absorbable and nonabsorbable) and severing of the nutrient artery during the osteotomy. The number of etiologies can be frustrating for the surgeon trying to maximize outcome and minimize potential complications. The use of advanced imaging techniques early in the postoperative course to identify the onset of AVN has further clouded the issue.

Austin and Leventen [21] and Johnson [23] reported no occurrence of AVN in their original studies, but Corless reported one case of AVN in his original study group. Other studies have followed, with the rate of occurrence ranging

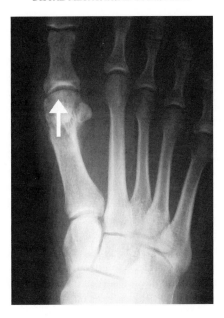

Fig. 14. Could this be AVN? Clinical correlation required.

from 0% to the Meier and Kenzora study, which noted a 40% rate of AVN with a chevron osteotomy and concomitant abductor release (Fig. 14) [37a].

In 1992, Wilkinson et al [38] used MRI to evaluate the formation of avascular necrosis following chevron bunionectomy. Their study was comprised of 25 bunionectomies; 20 were chevron bunionectomies with K-wire fixation and five were a control group of modified McBride bunionectomies. Using MRI between the fifth and twelfth postoperative weeks, they showed that 50% of the chevron bunionectomies presented a lesion on MRI consistent with AVN and that only 5% of these lesions presented on standard radiograph. Of the control group, none showed any signs of AVN. Though granting disruption of blood supply during any bunionectomy, these authors admit the main difference between chevron and control groups was a disruption of the main nutrient artery to the metatarsal. Their suggestion was to increase the plantar arm length and decrease the plantar first metatarsal and first interspace dissection to avoid disruption of blood supply. Though granting that MRI is more sensitive in the early detection of AVN lesions, Wilkinson et al [38] believe that these findings will probably not affect clinical outcome as the MRI changes did not result in statistically different clinical outcomes.

In a follow-up study in 1993, Neary et al [39] used MRI in the same fashion to study the potential onset of AVN in a patient group undergoing two different types of Austin bunionectomies. Four procedures were performed using what was deemed as the "anatomic technique," which consisted of a horizontally oriented medial flap of the joint capsule and a chevron osteotomy whose dorsal and plantar arms exited the cortex proximal to any synovial attachments. Eight procedures were described as the "angular technique," which was an inverted "L" medial capsule access while maintaining the classically described 60° angle of the osteotomy. Consistent to both procedures was that a lateral release was not performed on any patient. Only 1 of 12 revealed positive MRI changes consistent with AVN and it occurred with the anatomic technique. The authors of this study concluded that a lateral release with a chevron osteotomy significantly increases the risk of AVN, but they also concede that not performing a lateral release probably increases the chance of recurrence.

Later in 1993, Green et al [40] published a retrospective study of 164 procedures on 104 patients that underwent Austin bunionectomy with a lateral release. Of these, 148 were fixated with a single 2.7-mm screw and 16 with a single K-wire. These procedures were evaluated radiographically, with a mean follow-up of 30.4 months, and no evidence of AVN was found. An even larger retrospective study published in 1994 by Wallace et al [41] polled 45 surgeons that had trained at the same facility, resulting in a review of 13,952 DMOs. The review included Austin, Reverdin, Hohmann, Wilson, and Scarf osteotomies that were fixated with screw, pin, or absorbable rod. Only 15 procedures resulted in radiographic evidence of AVN, with 13 occurring in the Austin group. All reported incidences of AVN had undergone a lateral release. Green et al [40] found no increase in the rate of AVN when comparing types of fixation used. In 2002 Nery et al [29] studied 54 operative feet in 32 patients with an average follow-up of 2 years 11 months using the bicorrectional chevron osteotomy. They found no major complications, including no avascular necrosis. In 2003, Viehe et al [42] reported that in 95 chevron bunionectomies with screw fixation, 15 procedures experienced complications, none of which were AVN.

In the January 2004 *Podiatry Today*, Jeffrey Boberg, DPM, concisely reviews and organizes the debate on AVN and the DMO [43]. The authors echo his sentiments in that precise surgical technique is the deterrent for the formation of AVN, not omission of parts of the technique or even alteration of the osteotomy. The occurrence of AVN is probably higher than some of the later studies have shown, but it is likely that most occurrences are clinically insignificant. Though this subject warrants further study with more standardized research techniques, it is most important for the surgeon to recognize the early clinical signs of AVN and aggressively treat its onset.

Summary

Foot and ankle surgeons have a large and varied arsenal of osteotomies to correct the mild to moderate HAV deformity. The techniques for the various osteotomies have evolved over the years to allow the surgeon to match a procedure and its modifications to the individual patient's deformity, thus optimizing outcomes. Though some of the older osteotomies may still have a small faction of surgeons that prefer them, the authors believe that the chevron osteotomy remains at the forefront of mild to moderate HAV correction as it facilitates predictable results and affords the ability to modify the technique to fit the deformity present. Fixation techniques continue to evolve, and meticulous surgical technique to prevent complications remains a must. Regardless of the osteotomy used, the authors believe that adherence to the techniques laid out in today's literature will provide gratifying results for the surgeon and the patient.

References

[1] Hohmann G. Symptomatische oder physiologisch behandlung des hallux valgus. Munchen Med Wachnschr 1921;68:165–87.

[1a] Sanders AP, Snijders CJ, Linge BV. Potential for recurrence of hallux valgus after a modified Hohmann osteotomy: a biomechanical analysis. Foot Ankle 1995;16:351–6.

[2] Warrick JP, Edelman R. The Hohmann bunionectomy utilizing A-O screw fixation: a preliminary report. J Foot Surg 1984;23(4):268–74.

[3] Christensen PH, Hansen TB. Hallux valgus correction using a modified Hohmann technique. Foot Ankle Intl 1995;16(4):177–80.

[4] Heatherington V, editor. Hallux valgus and forefoot surgery. New York: Churchill Livingstone; 1994.

[5] Vogler HW. Shaft osteotomies in hallux valgus reduction. Clin Podiatr Med Surg 1989;6(1): 47–69.

[6] Peabody C. The surgical cure of hallux valgus. J Bone Joint Surg 1931;13:273.

[7] Hawkins FB, Mitchell CL, Hendrick DW. Correction of hallux valgus by metatarsal osteotomy. J Bone Joint Surg 1945;27(3):387.

[8] Blum JL. The modified Mitchell osteotomy-bunionectomy: indications and technical considerations. Foot Ankle Int 1994;15(3):103–6.

[9] Donovan JC. Results of bunion correction using Mitchell osteotomy. J Foot Surg 1982;21(3): 181–5.

[10] Teli M, et al. The Mitchell bunionectomy: a prospective study of 60 consecutive cases utilizing single K-wire fixation. J Foot Ankle Surg 2001;40(3):144–51.

[11] Wu KK. Mitchell bunionectomy: an analysis of four hundred and thirty personal cases plus a review of the literature. J Foot Surg 1987;26(4):277–92.

[11a] Weiner BK, Weiner DS, Mirkopulos N. Mitchell ostetomy for adolescent hallux valugus. J Pediatr Orthop 1997;17:781–4.

[11b] Forman WM, Cavolo DJ, Floyd EJ, et al. The Roux ostetomy: a correction for hallux abducto valgus deformity. J Am Podiatr Med Assoc 1984;74:596–600.

[12] Forman M, et al. The Roux osteotomy: a correction for hallux abducto valgus deformity. J Am Pod Assoc 1984;74(12):596–600.

[13] Wilson JN. Oblique displacement osteotomy for hallux valgus. J Bone Joint Surg [Br] 1963;45(3):552.

[14] Geldwert JJ, et al. Wilson bunionectomy with internal fixation: a ten-year experience. J Foot Surg 1991;30(6):574–9.

[14a] Helal B, Gupta SK, Gojosen P. Surgery for adolescent hallux valgus. Acta Orthop Scand 1974;45:271.

[14b] Klareskov B, Dalsgaard S, Gebuhr P. Wilson shaft osteotomy for hallux valgus. Acta Orthop Scand 1988;59:307–9.

[15] Grace D, Hughes J, Klenerman L. A comparison of Wilson and Hohmann osteotomies in the treatment of hallux valgus. J Bone Joint Surg [Br] 1988;70(2):236–41.

[15a] Allen TR, Gross M, Miller J, et al. The assessment of adolescent hallux valgus before and after first metatarsal osteotomy. Int Orthop 1981;5:111.

[16] White DL. Variations of the Wilson bunionectomy. Clin Podiatr Med Surg 1991;8(1):95–110.

[17] Reverdin J. De la deviation en dehors du gros orteil (hallux valgus, vulg. "Oignon bunions," "Ballen") et de son traitement chirurgical. Tr Internatl Med Congr 1881;2:408.

[18] Todd WF. Osteotomies of the first metatarsal head. Reverdin, Reverdin modifications, Peabody, Mitchell and Drato. In: Gerbert J, et al, editors. Textbook of bunion surgery. Mount Kisco (NY): Futura Publishing Co.; 1981.

[19] Zyzda MJ, Hineser W. Distal L osteotomy in treatment of hallux abducto valgus. J Foot Surg 1989;28(5):445.

[20] Lombardi CM, Silhanek AD, Connolly FG, et al. First metatarsocuneiform arthrodesis and Reverdin-Laird osteotomy for treatment of hallux valgus: an intermediate-term retrospective outcomes study. J Foot Ankle Surg 2003;42(2):77.

[21] Austin DW, Leventen EO. A new osteotomy for hallux valgus: a horizontally directed "V" displacement osteotomy of the metatarsal head for hallux valgus and primus varus. Clin Orthop Rel Res 1981;157:25.

[22] Corless JR. A modification of the Mitchell procedure [abstract]. J Bone Joint Surg [Br] 1976;58:138.

[23] Johnson KA, et al. Chevron osteotomy for hallux valgus. Clin Orthop Rel Res 1979;142:44.

[24] Velkes S, et al. Chevron osteotomy in the treatment of hallux valgus. J Foot Surg 1991; 30(3):276.

[25] Hetherington VJ, et al. The Austin bunionectomy: a follow-up study. J Foot Ankle Surg 1993;32(2):162.

[26] Bar-David T, et al. A retrospective analysis of distal chevron and basilar osteotomies of the first metatarsal for correction of intermetatarsal angles in the range of 13 to 16 degrees. J Foot Surg 1991;30(5):450.

[27] Steinstra JJ, et al. Large displacement distal chevron osteotomy for the correction of hallux valgus deformity. J Foot Ankle Surg 2002;41(4):213.

[28] Gerbert J, et al. Bi-correctional horizontal v-osteotomy (Austin-type) of the first metatarsal head. J Am Podiatry Assoc 1979;69(2):119.

[29] Nery C, et al. Biplanar chevron osteotomy. Foot Ankle Int 2002;23(9):792.

[30] Youngwick FD. Modifications of the Austin bunionectomy for treatment of metatarsus primus elevatus associated with hallux limitus. J Foot Surgery 1982;21(2):114.

[31] Gerbert J, et al. Youngswick-Austin procedure: the effect of plantar arm orientation on metatarsal head displacement. J Foot Ankle Surg 2001;41(1):8.

[32] Kalish SR. Modifications of the Austin hallux valgus repair (Kalish osteotomy). In: McGlamry ED, editor. Reconstructive surgery of the foot and leg—update '89. Tucker (GA): Podiatry Institute; 1989. p. 14–9.

[33] Kalish SR. The Kalish osteotomy. A review and retrospective analysis of 265 cases. J Am Podiatr Med Assoc 1994;84(5):237.

[34] Downey MS. Complications of the Kalish bunionectomy. J Am Podiatr Med Assoc 1994; 84(5):243.

[35] Khuri J, et al. Fixation of the offset V osteotomy: mechanical testing of 4 constructs. J Foot Ankle Surg 2003;42(2):63–7.

[35a] Ludloff K. Die Beseitigung des Hallux valgus durch die schraege planto-dorsale osteotomie des metatarsus I. Arch Klin Chir 1918;110:364–87.

[36] Dalton S, et al. Stability of the offset V osteotomy: effects of fixation, orientation and surgical translocation in polyurethane foam models and preserved cadaveric specimens. J Foot Ankle Surg 2003;42(2):53–62.

[36a] Fox IM, Cuttic M, De Marco P. The offset V modification of the chevron bunionectomy: a retrospective study. J Foot Surgery 1992 Nov–Dec;31(6):615–20.

[36b] Shereff MJ, Sobel MA, Kummer FJ. The stability of fixation of first metatarsal osteotomies. Foot Ankle 1991 Feb;11(4):208–11.

[36c] Landsman AS, Voger HW. An assessment of oblique base wedge osteotomy stability in the first metatarsal using different modes of internal fixation. J Foot Surg 1992 May–Jun;31(3):211–8.

[36d] Buckenberger RK, Goldman FD. Chevron bunionectomy fixation, in vitro stability assess-

ment of plate-and-screw system compared with Kirschner wire. J Foot And Ankle Surg 1995 May–June;34(3):266–72.

[36e] Chang T, Landsman AS, Ruch JA. Relative strengths of internal fixation in osteotomies and arthrodesis of the first metatarsal in reconstructive surgery of the foot and leg: Update 1996. Tucker, GA: Podiatry Institute Publishing; 1992. p. 120–7.

[37] Jacobson K, et al. Mechanical comparison of fixation techniques for the offset V osteotomy: a saw bone study. J Foot Ankle Surg 2003;42(6):339–43.

[37a] Kenzora JE, Meier PJ. The risks and benefits of distal first metatarsal osteotomy. Foot Ankle 1985;6:7–17.

[38] Wilkinson SV, et al. Austin bunionectomy: postoperative MRI evaluation for avascular necrosis. J Foot Surg 1992;31(5):469–77.

[39] Neary M, et al. Avascular necrosis of the first metatarsal head following Austin osteotomy: a follow-up study. J Foot Surg 1993;32(5):530–5.

[40] Green M, et al. Avascular necrosis following distal chevron osteotomy of the first metatarsal. J Foot Ankle Surg 1993;31(6):617–22.

[41] Wallace G, et al. Avascular necrosis following distal first metatarsal osteotomies: a survey. J Foot Ankle Surg 1994;33(2):167–72.

[42] Viehe R, et al. Complications of screw-fixated chevron osteotomies for the correction hallux abducto valgus. JAPMA 2003;93(6):499–502.

[43] Boberg J. Avascular necrosis after bunion surgery. Podiatry Today January 2004:28–34.

ELSEVIER
SAUNDERS

Clin Podiatr Med Surg
22 (2005) 169–195

CLINICS IN
PODIATRIC
MEDICINE AND
SURGERY

Midshaft First-Ray Osteotomies for Hallux Valgus

Matthew S. Rockett, DPM, FACFAS[a],*, Larry R. Goss, DPM, FACFAS, FACFAOM[b]

[a]Bay Area Podiatry Associates, 1234 Bay Area Boulevard, Suite G, Houston, TX 77058, USA
[b]Temple University School of Podiatric Medicine, 8th at Race Streets,
Philadelphia, PA 19107-2496, USA

Surgical techniques and procedure selection for painful hallux valgus deformity runs the gamut of various techniques and philosophies. Over 140 different procedures have been described in the literature, ranging from simple exostectomy to arthrodesis of the first metatarsophalangeal joint. This article describes the two most common shaft osteotomies performed for the correction of hallux valgus: the offset V osteotomy and Z osteotomy.

Shaft osteotomies are defined as those procedures that incise cortical bone almost entirely in the diaphysis of the first metatarsal. In the past, shaft osteotomies were avoided because of the belief that these osteotomies disrupted the blood supply to the first metatarsal and that this could lead to complications in healing. Furthermore, this type of osteotomy was more technically demanding when compared with the more popular distal metaphyseal procedures. With the improvement of osteosynthesis to stabilize the osteotomy, shaft procedures were described to correct bunion deformities with higher intermetatarsal angles that the distal capital osteotomies could not correct.

History

Numerous modifications of the distal chevron osteotomy have been reported. One of its variations, the offset V osteotomy, came from a modification of the

---

* Corresponding author.
E-mail address: rockettman@houston.rr.com (M.S. Rockett).

0891-8422/05/$ – see front matter © 2005 Elsevier Inc. All rights reserved.
doi:10.1016/j.cpm.2004.11.004

podiatric.theclinics.com

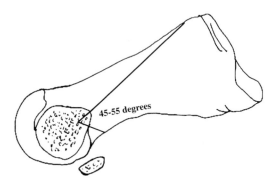

Fig. 1. Lateral offset V bunionectomy diagram depicting the long dorsal arm of 4.0 to 5.0 cm and short plantar wing with an angle of 45 to 55 degrees.

distal 60-degree chevron osteotomy. Two authors are credited with the development and popularization of this change in the osteotomy placement—Harold Vogler [1] and Stanley Kalish [2]. These authors moved the apex of the osteotomy to the proximal margin of the metaphyseal region and created an osteotomy with an apex angled from 45 to 55 degrees. Entirely placed within diaphyseal bone of the metatarsal, the dorsal cut of the offset V is at least 4.0 to 5.0 cm proximally directed (Fig. 1). This long dorsal arm provides three advantages over the distal metaphyseal osteotomy. First, the osteotomy may be transposed as much as 50% of the first metatarsal as compared with the distal osteotomies because of the larger surface area of bone contact. Second, because of the larger surface area, two points of rigid internal fixation could be used to stabilize the osteotomy. Additionally, because of the interlocking nature of the osteotomy, it is inherently stable.

Z osteotomy

In 1926, Meyer [3] first described the principle of the "Z bunionectomy" technique in search for greater stability of the corrective first metatarsal osteotomies. At this time, the use of this operative technique was limited secondary to lack of sophisticated osteotomy instrumentation, limited internal fixation methods, and poor understanding of the osteotomy design. Fifty years later, in 1976, Burutaran [4] presented a series of four cases where a Z procedure, in combination with a Keller bunionectomy, was performed for the correction of hallux valgus deformity.

In 1983, after having critically analyzed the Mau osteotomy, Charles Gudas developed the modern Z osteotomy (Fig. 2). The Z osteotomy evolved from the Mau osteotomy, which is also a shaft osteotomy but rarely used today. The basis for the Mau osteotomy was to use the strong dorsal cortex and transpose the plantar capital fragment laterally. Zygmunt, Gudas, and Laros [5] described the Z osteotomy in the literature in 1989 depicting three interlocking cuts in the diaphyseal bone of the first metatarsal with a long horizontal cut in through the

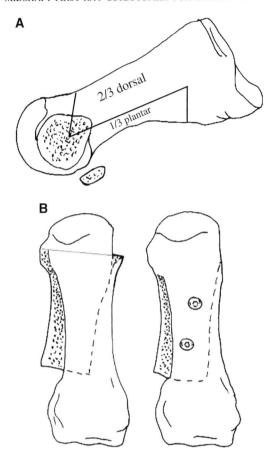

Fig. 2. (*A*) Lateral view of the Z osteotomy. It is important that the cut is made in a two-thirds dorsal and one-third plantar ratio. (*B*) Dorsoplantar view of the Z-osteotomy diagram.

first metatarsal. Like the offset V osteotomy, this osteotomy provided significantly more lateral translation and surface area than the distal osteotomies and provided for the application of rigid internal osteosynthesis using a lag technique because of the strong dorsal cortex of the metatarsal. Secondary to the strength of the internal fixation of both osteotomies, immediate weight bearing postoperatively by the patient was possible without casting.

In 1984, Borrelli and Weil [7] gave the name "scarf" to this bunionectomy technique from a carpentry term for "a joint made by notching, grooving, or beveling two beams and fastening them together so that they lap over and join firmly into one continuous piece." Their contribution to the osteotomy included modifying the cuts, increasing the length, and studying the blood supply in regards to the osteotomies. The "short Z bunionectomy" was first described in 1986 by Glickman and Zahari [8]. In 1994, Miller et al [9], using matched paired cadaveric specimens, described the inverted Z bunionectomy.

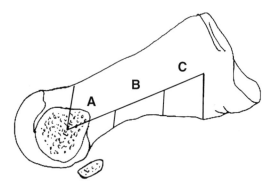

Fig. 3. Diagram showing the three levels of the Z bunionectomy. (*A*) Short Z; (*B*) medium Z; (*C*) long Z bunionectomy.

Louis Barouk is credited with popularizing the Z-type procedure in France and Europe. He has performed over 3000 scarf bunionectomies, and his contributions include displacement of the osteotomy, lowering the first metatarsal head, shortening the first ray, and different internal fixation methods [10–12]. Shortening as proposed by Barouk is performed for two reasons: to provide longitudinal decompression of the first ray and to preserve the MTP joint range of motion. Barouk has additionally designed a specific "scarf screw" that has a self-tapping, threaded head to provide compression [10]. He applies the distal screw in a 45-degree angle into the metatarsal head. Many modifications exist for the Z bunionectomy [13–16]. It may be performed as a short Z (IM angle of 13 degrees or less), a medium Z (IM angle of 14 to 16 degrees), and a long Z for (IM angle of 17 to 19 degrees) (Fig. 3). Several authors have advocated that the procedure may be performed on higher IM angles; however, there is a higher likelihood of potential undercorrection and recurrence if the metatarsal is narrow or hypermobility exists [10,12]. In this article, the authors describe the indications; contraindications; surgical technique and its fixation considerations; postoperative care; results; and potential complications of the offset V and the traditional Z osteotomies.

Indications

Moderate-to-severe structural hallux abductovalgus deformity may be treated with shaft osteotomies (Box 1) (Fig. 4). There are no age limits for these procedures; however, caution should be used with severe juvenile hallux abductovalgus, as the growth plate is proximal at the base of the first metatarsal in this patient population and the osteotomy should not enter the growth plate. There should be a congruous joint with pain-free range of motion. Range of motion should be greater than 40 degrees of the first MTP joint. Bone density should be adequate to support internal fixation. Increased PASA (proximal

---

Box 1. Indications for shaft osteotomies

Intermetatarsal angle of 12 to 19 degrees
PASA deformity less than 14 degrees
Range of motion greater than 40 degrees
No joint arthrosis
Hallux abductus angle greater than 15 degrees
Normal or long metatarsal protrusion distance
Tibial sesamoidal position less than 6
Adequate bone stock
No hypermobility of the first metatarsocuneiform joint

---

articular set angle) and DMAA (distal metatarsal articular angle) of less than 14 degrees may be corrected with rotation of these osteotomies (see references [1,2,5–8,10,12–25]).

Contraindications

Though there are few absolute contraindications for the Z bunionectomy, the authors propose the following as a guide (Table 1).

Surgical technique

Operative dissection for the Z and offset V osteotomies are identical. Two skin incisions are commonly employed to approach the first metatarsal, either a

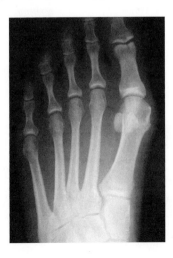

Fig. 4. AP radiograph of a moderate structural bunion deformity with no arthrosis of the first metatarsophalangeal joint. This type of deformity is ideal for the use of a shaft osteotomy.

Table 1
Contraindication for the shaft osteotomies

Absolute contraindications	Relative contraindications
Hypermobility of the first ray	ROM less than 30 degrees
Arthrosis of the first MTPJ	Osteoporosis
Vascular compromise	Elderly patient (greater than 70 years old)
Severe metatarsus primus varus (IM angle greater than 20 degrees)	Obesity
Severe metatarsus primus elevatus	Short first ray
	Narrow first metatarsal (Z bunionectomy)
	Non-compliance

dorsomedial or medial incision. The dorsomedial incision is made longitudinally and is 5 to 7 cm in length. This incision is made halfway between the high point of the medial eminence of the first metatarsal head and the extensor hallucis longus tendon centered over the shaft and head of the first metatarsal. With the medial incision, it is created by outlining the first metatarsal head, and the 5- to 7-cm longitudinal incision is placed bisecting the outline of the metatarsal head and shaft (Fig. 5). The decision to use either incision is typically based on the size of the deformity and cosmesis. Medial incisions typically have better cosmesis, but can only be used on patients with smaller intermetatarsal angles or where minimal lateral releases need to be performed.

Dissection through the subcutaneous layer is performed taking care to protect and retract the medial neurovascular structures. Subsequently, the capsule of the first metatarsophalangeal joint is identified. When using a dorsomedial incision, the contracted lateral metatarsophalangeal structures are released first, versus the medial incision where the capsulotomy is performed first. These

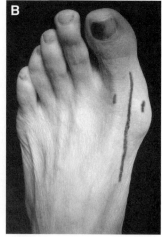

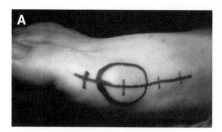

Fig. 5. The two incisional approaches for shaft osteotomies. (*A*) Medial incision; (*B*) Dorso-medial incision.

structures include the fibular sesamoidal ligament, lateral capsule of the first metatarsophalangeal joint, and the oblique and transverse heads of the adductor hallucis tendon. This is performed by development of a subcutaneous tissue plane on the lateral side of the joint and placing a self-retaining retractor to protect the extensor tendons medially and the skin laterally. Caution is taken not to overzealously release the joint or cut the lateral head of the flexor hallucis brevis. Our rationale to release the lateral capsule first is that by cutting the contracted structures before performing a medial capsulotomy, you can be assured that the structures that you are cutting are under maximal contracture versus after the capsulotomy and periosteal elevation when some laxity can be afforded to these structures.

After the lateral release is completed, the capsulotomy and periosteal elevation is performed. The authors use two converging semielliptical incisions made over the high point of the medial eminence, and the capsule is excised. However, various other types of capsular incisions may be performed based on surgeons' preference. An incision is then made from the proximal apex of the capsulotomy in the periosteum along the medial aspect of the first metatarsal shaft to the level of the proximal metaphyseal flare. A landmark for this periosteal incision is the extensor hallucis capsularis. Periosteal incisional placement should be 1 to 2 mm medial to the extensor hallucis capsularis so that the incision is not too close to the extensor hallucis longus tendon and there is not enough periosteum to close over the metatarsal shaft. After this is performed, the capsule and periosteum are sharply dissected by use of a scalpel and periosteal elevator to expose the first metatarsal shaft dorsally and plantarly to facilitate performing the osteotomies.

Next, the medial eminence is resected using a sagittal saw. This prominence is cut parallel to the first metatarsal shaft so that there is no extra bony shelf plantarly that can cause potential tyloma formation in the future. Care is taken that the medial sesamoidal groove is not disrupted. Therefore, at least 2 mm should be left on the metatarsal head medial to the tibial sesamoidal groove (Fig. 6). If using a medial incision, the lateral release is performed retracting

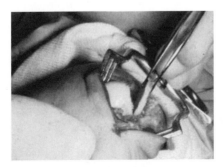

Fig. 6. Resection of the medial eminence is performed 2 mm medial to the medial sagittal groove of the first metatarsal end. Preservation of the medial sagittal groove is paramount to prevent potential hallux varus.

the plantar capsule and placing a scalpel under the metatarsal head and through the joint to release the lateral contracted structures. After these steps are completed, the osteotomies are ready to be performed.

Zosteotomy surgical technique

Though other authors have modified the Z osteotomy cuts and given it different names, such as scarf, rotational, short and inverted, the authors still perform the osteotomy cuts as originally described by Zygmunt, Gudas, and Laros in 1983 and published in 1989 [5]. The Z osteotomy consists of three bone cuts performed in the following order: central/horizontal, distal/dorsal, and proximal/plantar. First, the osteotomy is drawn on the medial side of the first metatarsal (Fig. 7). The central horizontal arm extends from approximately 1.0 to 1.5 cm proximal to the articular surface of the metatarsal head to 2 to 3 cm from the proximal metaphyseal flare. As a general rule, the length of the horizontal cut should be at least twice the width of the metatarsal shaft. This will allow adequate shift of the capital fragment and permit two points of internal fixation. It is also extremely important when drawing the osteotomy that this horizontal line divides the metatarsal into two-thirds dorsally and one-third plantarly. This is essential to prevent and dorsal stress risers at the proximal osteotomy site.

From the horizontal central line, the dorsal limb is drawn to form a 70-degree angle with the horizontal line. This dorsal line is carried onto the top of the metatarsal. It is paramount that this line is perpendicular to the second metatarsal, not the first metatarsal. If this is not perpendicular to the second metatarsal, the osteotomy may not translate laterally after completing the osteotomy. Proximally the plantar arm is then drawn creating another 70-degree angle.

After the lines have been drawn on the bone, the osteotomy is now performed. Using a small bone saw, the horizontal bone cut completed is first. When making this cut it is crucial that the cut be made at a 10 to 15 degree angle plantarly from medial to lateral in relation to the transverse plane of the first metatarsal and

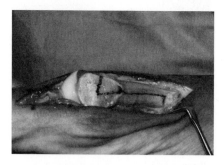

Fig. 7. Intraoperative drawing of the proposed Z-osteotomy site.

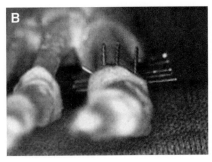

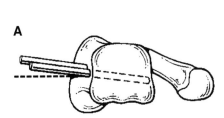

Fig. 8. (*A*) Diagram showing 10- to 15-degree angle plantarly from medial to lateral in relation to the transverse plane of the first metatarsal and weight-bearing surface for the horizontal cut of the Z osteotomy. (*B*) Frontal plane relationship of the horizontal cut of the Z osteotomy a saw bone model with the k wires representing no plantar angulation.

weight-bearing surface (Fig. 8). To gauge this angle, the forefoot is loaded into the neutral position with the surgeon's hand that is not holding the saw (Fig. 9). By doing this, the surgeon can determine the amount of plantar angulation to establish in relation to the contralateral hand, which is mimicking the weight-bearing surface. After the horizontal cut is completed, the dorsal distal cut is next. Using the same saw blade, this cut is made perpendicular to the second metatarsal. It is essential when making this cut that the saw blade does not over cut plantarly beyond the horizontal cut, which can produce a stress riser at the metatarsal head level. Lastly, the proximal plantar cut is created. Using a narrower saw blade, this cut is made either parallel to the distal cut or angle 5 to 10 degrees proximal lateral to allow for any PASA correction by swiveling the proximal cut.

Once the cuts are performed and the plantar capital fragment is free, the capital fragment is transposed laterally over one-third to one-half the width of the first metatarsal. Temporary fixation in the form of a bone reduction forceps is used to hold the corrected position (Fig. 10). While applying the bone reduc-

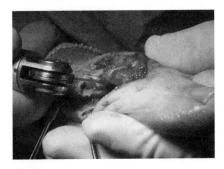

Fig. 9. Intraoperatively, the forefoot is loaded with the hand opposite of the saw to gauge the angle of the cut.

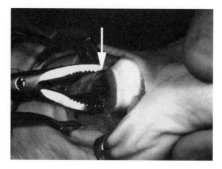

Fig. 10. After the osteotomy is translated laterally, a bone reduction forceps is used to temporarily hold the osteotomy.

tion forceps, it is critical to make sure that the surgeon does not apply too much pressure or that any troughing is noted. If troughing is seen, the osteotomy must be slight shifted to allow for more bone contact or bone graft added. Troughing will be discussed in more detail in the complications section. The correction of the deformity is subsequently verified clinically and radiographically. Internal fixation of osteotomy is performed using two points of fixation. Fixation techniques for the osteotomies are discussed later in the section on fixation considerations.

Offset V surgical technique

A V-shaped osteotomy [1,2] with apex directed distally is placed completely through the first metatarsal head. The apex of the osteotomy is at the periphery of an imaginary circle and the angulation between the dorsal and plantar arms is approximately 45 to 55 degrees (Fig. 11). Intraoperatively, the osteotomy is drawn on the medial side of the first metatarsal. From the apex mark, the short arm extends plantarly and proximally 1.0 to 1.5 cm in length to exit behind the sesamoidal complex. The long dorsal arm is directed proximally and superiorly 4.0 to 5.0 cm (varies depending on the length of the first metatarsal) and should

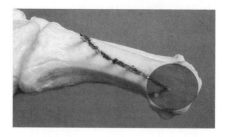

Fig. 11. Depiction of offset V osteotomy on a saw bone model. Note the proximal location of the apex at the periphery of the imaginary circle (*darkened circle*).

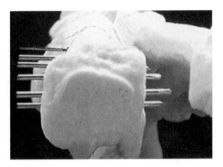

Fig. 12. Saw bone model demonstrating the angulation of the offset V osteotomy, which is oriented with zero degrees of angulation.

be long enough to accommodate two cortical screws, as well as exit before the proximal metaphyseal/diaphyseal junction of the first metatarsal. Care must be taken with the long dorsal cut to avoid inadvertent violation into the first metatarsal-cuneiform joint proximally [1,2].

The first cut performed is the dorsal long arm. Using an appropriately sized saw blade, the dorsal arm is cut with the saw blade parallel to the floor or zero degrees plantar angulation. It is essential that the cut is made with zero-degree angulation so that the osteotomy does not over plantarflex or dorsiflex (Fig. 12). If the dorsal arm appears to be exiting too proximally, the osteotomy may be notched perpendicular to dorsal cortex to complete the cut. After the dorsal arm is completed, the plantar arm is cut using a small saw blade. Unlike the Z osteotomy, this cut is made perpendicular to the first metatarsal and not the second metatarsal. If the cut is made more perpendicular to the second metatarsal, the osteotomy will jam proximally when transposing the osteotomy.

The capital fragment is displaced laterally upon the proximal fragment approximately 30% to 50% of the width of the first metatarsal shaft. If significant deviation of the proximal articular set angle is noted intraoperatively, then the capital fragment can be rotated medially to correct for this deformity by first overcorrecting the intermetatarsal angle and then swiveling at the proximal apex. Temporary fixation and imaging is then employed similar to the Z bunionectomy and then stabilized with two points of fixation.

Fixation considerations

After the osteotomies are completed, two points of fixation are needed to secure these osteotomies to allow for primary bone healing and stability of the fractures. Originally, the fixation for the Z bunionectomy was either two 3.5-mm or 2.7-mm cortical screws. Offset V-osteotomy fixation was initially described as either a single 0.062 K-wire or two 2.7-mm screws. With time and the evolution of different fixation techniques, other techniques have been described.

Table 2
Different fixation constructs

One or two 2.7-mm Synthes screws	Two Barouk screw or Herbert screws
Two 2.0-mm Synthes screws	One 0.062 inch K-wire
Two 2.4-mm Synthes screws (Authors' Preference)	Two 3.5-mm Synthes screws
Two 2.4-mm Osteomed MX screws	Orthosorb pins
One 2.7 mm and one 2.0 mm Synthes screw	Allograft cortical pins
One 2.7-mm and one threaded or smooth K-wire (0.062, 0.045, or 0.035 inch)	Trimet screws

Listed in Table 2 are some of the different fixation constructs that have been described (see references [1,2,5,9,10,12–28]).

There are many options the surgeon has for fixating these osteotomies. In designing the fixation construct to be used for these osteotomies, the surgeon must take into account what fixation is best for the patient, which fixation is the strongest with the least potential of complication, and what fixation the surgeon feels most comfortable using. With all of the fixation options possible, one underlying principle needs to be followed, that being the osteotomies must be fixated with two points of fixation to decrease complications. Downey [18], when analyzing the complications of the Kalish offset V osteotomy, suggested that when the osteotomies are rigidly fixated with two points of fixation that the complications were significantly reduced.

Fox et al [19] retrospectively compared single K-wire fixation versus screw fixation and found that the results indicated that both produce similar outcomes. However, they concluded that there appears to be many advantages to screw fixation over K-wire fixation. They found when using screws, the result was rigid internal fixation and primary bone healing. When compared with K-wire fixation, which does not result in rigid fixation, there was secondary bone healing and a greater risk of motion at the osteotomy site with prolonged postoperative edema due to the motion. Additionally, screw fixation allows an earlier return to range of motion of the first metatarsophalangeal joint by allowing the patient into a soft shoe at 3 weeks.

Friend et al [13] analyzed 54 Z bunionectomies were performed on 43 patients. Twenty-nine osteotomies were fixated with OrthoSorb (Johnson & Johnson, Piscataway, New Jersey) pins, and 25 were fixated with a single 2.7-mm. cortical screw. They found that the incidence of first metatarsal head dorsiflexion in screw fixated osteotomies was double that of OrthoSorb. Two patients with OrthoSorb had dislocation of the capital fragment and had to be refixated. Radiographic evidence of pin tracts persisted beyond 1 year in about half the OrthoSorb-fixated osteotomies. However, the authors concluded that in properly selected patients, OrthoSorb is as effective as a screw in fixating the osteotomy.

Kissel, Unroe, and Parker [20] described the use of one 2.7-mm screw and one buried 0.035-inch K-wire in the offset V osteotomy. Initially the authors used two-screw fixation for the osteotomy, but they found that the thin cortex of the capital fragment proximally was often inadequate for optimal countersinking of the screw and caused fracture of the proximal screw when tightened. No fractures were reported, but 15% required removal of the fixation.

In 2003, four studies were published on testing the mechanical strength of these osteotomies. Jacobson et al [26] tested four different techniques for the fixation of an offset V bunionectomy were on solid-foam saw-bone models for the purpose of determining the strongest form of fixation for the osteotomy. These techniques were group 1 (two 2.7-mm cortical screws), group 2 (one 2.7-mm cortical screw and one 2.0-mm cortical screw), group 3 (two 2.0-mm cortical screws), and group 4 (one 2.7-mm cortical screw and one 0.062-inch threaded k-wire). Their results showed the mean force to failure of the groups was group 1, 58.1 N; group 2, 59.3 N; group 3, 64.0 N; and group 4, 105.66 N. There was a statistical significant difference between group 4 and the other three groups. There was no statistical difference between groups 1 to 3. In groups 1 to 3, 87% of the failures were through the distal screw hole, whereas the remaining 13% were through the proximal screw hole. In group 4, 60% of the failures were through the proximal fixation point and 40% were through the distal screw hole (Fig. 13). We concluded that, in this model, the strongest form of fixation for an offset

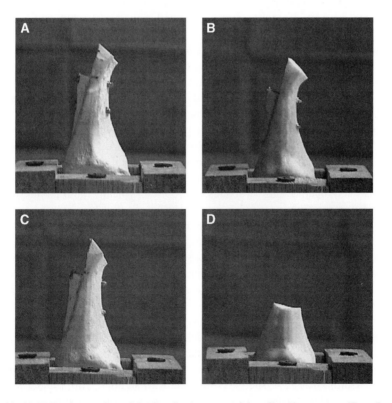

Fig. 13. (*A–D*) Breakage points of the four fixation types of the offset V osteotomy. (*From* Jacobson K, Gough A, Mendicino SS, Rockett MS. Mechanical comparison of fixation techniques for the offset V osteotomy: a sawbone study. J Foot Ankle Surg 2003;42:339–43.)

V osteotomy was the 2.7-mm cortical screw placed distally with the proximal point of fixation being a threaded 0.062-inch Kirschner wire.

Khuri et al [27] did a similar study in which they tested four forms of fixation constructs and a control using the same types of models as Jacobson et al [26]. In their study, they tested two 2.0-mm cortical screws, two 2.7-mm cortical screws, and two 3.5-mm cortical screws in the offset V osteotomy. Their results differed from Jacobson in two areas. First the area of fracture or failure was proximal to the fixation devices not through the fixation sites as seen in our study. Also they found that there was no statistically significant difference in the maximum load sustained by the test fixation groups. They concluded that all fixation techniques were equal in strength and that any of the constructs may be used for the fixation of the osteotomy.

Dalton et al [28] tested the stability of the offset V first metatarsal osteotomy in polyurethane foam models and cadaver specimens. In their study they tested the effect of lateral translation of the osteotomy and orientation of the fixation. Their results revealed that using plantar wing K-wire orientation showed statistically significantly greater stiffness and load at failure than the dorsal wing-pin orientation group in saw bones. Cadaveric offset V specimens received the same amount of capital fragment lateral translocation but had different fixation types and orientations. The cadaveric dorsal wing-screw group showed statistically significantly less displacement at failure than the plantar wing-screw, plantar wing-pin, and dorsal wing-pin groups. The dorsal wing-pin group with a synthetic tension band showed a statistically significant greater stiffness and peak load at failure compared with the dorsal wing-pin group without the tension band. The most stable offset V construct in the polyurethane foam model was the plantar wing-pin group. However, preserved cadaveric specimens yielded different results. The cadaveric dorsal wing-pin group with the synthetic tension band showed superior stability compared with all other non–tension-band groups. These results indicate the importance of tension band effects provided by capsular and ligamentous structures, which are typically ignored in surgical optimization research.

Popoff et al [29] tested the effect of screw types on the biomechanical properties of a modified Z osteotomy (SCARF) and crescentic osteotomies using a cannulated Barouk 3-mm screw and a solid core 4.0-mm cancellous screw in a cadaveric study. They found that the in the Z osteotomy type that the Barouk screws were stiffer compared with the cancellous screws, but this difference was not statistically significant. The Z-type osteotomy was statistically stronger than the fixation for the crescentic osteotomy. Failure for the fixation of the Z-type osteotomy was different in that the cancellous screw failed at the bony bridge and the Barouk screw failed by screw migration.

In selecting fixation for these osteotomies, it is important that the surgeon selects fixation that he or she is comfortable with and that will promote primary bone healing and resistance to rotation. The authors have tried many different forms of fixation, but their preference for fixation of these osteotomies is either two 2.7-mm cortical screws or two 2.4-mm cortical AO screws (Fig. 14). The

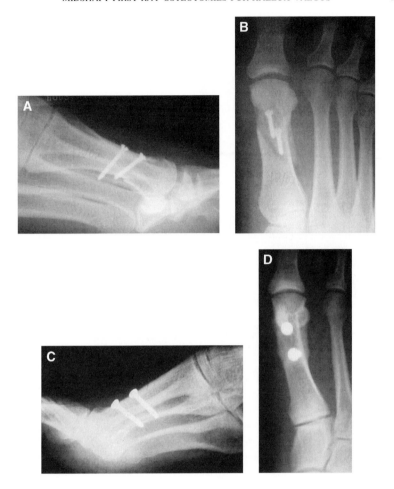

Fig. 14. (*A–D*) Radiographs of an offset V osteotomy fixated with two 2.4-mm cortical screws. (*A*) Lateral; (*B*) AP. Radiographs of a Z osteotomy fixated with two 2.7-mm cortical screws. (*C*) Lateral; (*D*) AP.

2.4-mm screw is preferred by the authors because it has a lower profile head and is self-tapping, which eliminates a step in screw insertion and therefore decreases the stress that is being applied to the osteotomy. Each screw is placed perpendicular to osteotomy in standard AO/ASIF technique. It is essential that you do not overcountersink or go too deep with the overdrill. If you excessively countersink, a stress riser may develop in the dorsal cortex. If you penetrate too far with the overdrill, the screw may not afford compression by loss of the lag effect of the screw and may necessitate having to use a large screw.

Besides being perpendicular to the osteotomy, there are two other important aspects to remember placing the screws. First, one must resist placing the screws too close together. If the screws are too close together you can develop a stress

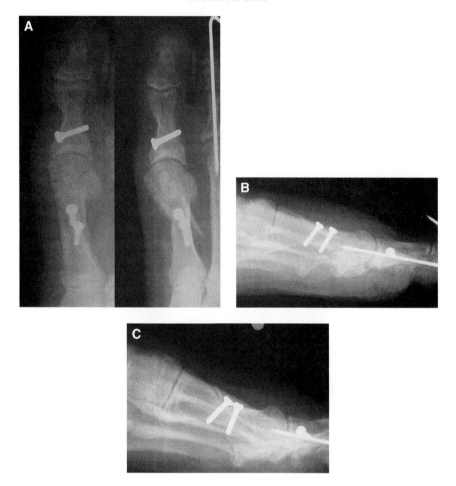

Fig. 15. (*A*) AP radiographs of an offset V osteotomy with 2.7-mm screws placed too close to-gether. The radiograph on the left is immediate postoperatively and 1 week after the patient started walking on the foot. (*B*) Lateral radiograph immediately postoperatively. Note that the screws are placed too close together and the proximal screw is placed too close to the proximal end of the osteotomy. (*C*) Fracture of the osteotomy between the screw and proximal to the proximal screw.

riser and fracture the dorsal wing (Fig. 15). Second, it is important to avoid the "no-fly zones" as proposed by the authors (Fig. 16). If a screw is placed in any of these zones, one of two things can occur—either distraction of the osteotomy site with loss of compression or fracture of the osteotomy.

After the fixation is complete, the overhanging medial bone is resected flush with the metatarsal shaft and a rotary bur is used to smooth any rough edges. It is recommended at this point that the foot be reimaged and manually loaded to determine if any ancillary phalangeal osteotomies need to be performed.

Deep capsular closure is performed using a 2-0 absorbable suture. It is important that when the periosteal capsular layer is being repaired an assistant

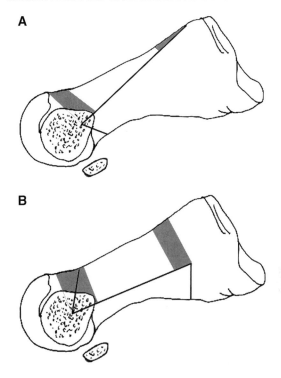

Fig. 16. Depiction of "no-fly zones" as represented by the darkened areas on the drawing. Screws placed into these areas can create fracturing of the osteotomy. (*A*) Offset V; (*B*) Z osteotomy.

or surgical technician is holding the hallux in a rectus and plantarflexed position. If the toe is not held plantarflexed, the patient may have problems with hallux purchase after the surgery. After the capsule is repaired, the subcutaneous tissue is subsequently closed with an absorbable 4-0 suture. Skin closure is performed using the surgeon's preference; however, the authors' preferred technique is using a subcitular stitch with an absorbable monofilament 4-0 suture and steristrips (Fig. 17). Upon completion of the procedure, a dry, sterile compressive dressing with the toe splinted in neutral is applied.

Postoperative care

Immediately postoperatively, the patient is placed in either a surgical shoe or a removable cast boot and instructed remain non–weight bearing for 2 weeks. Originally, both procedures were designed and described to allow for immediate postoperative ambulation in a surgical shoe to permit bathroom and other essential activities of daily living. Until recently, this was the typical postoperative protocol for the authors. The authors have found that placing the patient non-weight bearing for a 2-week period substantially reduces postoperative

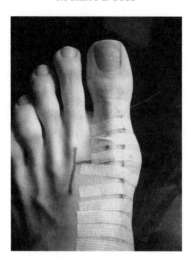

Fig. 17. Closure of the dorsomedial skin incision with absorbable suture and steri-strips.

pain and edema. The patient is usually given oral antibiosis for 3 days and anti-inflammatory medication for 2 weeks along with narcotic analgesics. The patient is also instructed to elevate the operative foot on two pillows and apply ice 2 hours on then 2 hours off for the first 72 hours. At week 1 postoperatively, the patient returns to clinic or office for a dressing change and postoperative foot radiographs (AP and lateral). A smaller compressive dressing is applied and the patient is again instructed to remain non-weight bearing and scheduled for a follow-up in 1 week. It is important to keep the hallux in proper neutral alignment during the dressing changes and to refrain from overcorrecting the hallux into a varus position.

During the second postoperative visit, depending on the suture technique employed, sutures are removed or the ends of the subcuticular suture are trimmed flush with the skin. Another compressive dressing is applied, and the patient is instructed on passive range-of-motion exercises. These exercises are useful to help restore the range of motion and decrease postoperative stiffness. Each patient is instructed to hold the foot stable at the metatarsocuneiform joint with the ipsilateral hand and apply the thumb and index finger of the contralateral hand to hold the hallux at the interphalangeal joint and maximally dorsiflex and plantarflex the hallux until they feel discomfort and hold for 10 seconds. It is essential that the patient grasp the hallux at the interphalangeal joint and not the tip of the hallux to ensure proper stretching of the first metatarsophalangeal joint. This exercise is to be performed three times a day performing 10 repetitions. Weight bearing is typically permitted at this point in the surgical shoe, and the patient is reappointed for 1 week.

Three weeks postoperatively another series of radiographs are taken of the foot and if there are no changes in the position the patient is instructed to start ambulating in a gym shoe or other soft lace-up shoe. At this point, the patient is permitted to bathe the foot and apply lotion or creams to reduce any potential scar formation. Additionally, the patient is dispensed and instructed on the use of either 4-inch coban (3M Corporation) or Surgi-grip to help reduce edema. Range-of-motion exercises are stressed again and are to be continued by the patient. If the right foot was operated on, the patient is instructed that they can start driving if they are wearing the gym shoe comfortably all day and that pressure on the brake and gas pedal does not provide any discomfort. The patient is scheduled for follow-up in 3 weeks.

At 6 weeks, the patient again has radiographs taken to determine if the osteotomy has healed. If the patient is pain-free in their gym shoes, they are advanced into dress shoes and heels as tolerated. It is stressed to the patient that they should always have a back-up pair of shoes with them in case the shoes they are wearing start feeling uncomfortable. Range of motion of the first meta-tarsophalangeal joint is reevaluated and if the patient's range of motion is within normal limits they are instructed to stop the exercises. If the range of motion is inadequate or stiffness is present, the patient is instructed to continue home range of motion exercises or sent for a course of formal physical therapy. Exercise in the form of aquatic or stationary bike is now permitted. The patient is scheduled at 6 more weeks, and at that visit is usually discharged and allowed to start normal exercise activities as tolerated.

Results of the osteotomies in the literature

Kalish and Spector [2], in 1984, reported on a sample from their initial 265 offset V osteotomies. They found that osteotomy significantly and adequately reduced the intermetatarsal angle and hallux abductus angle with predictable and reliable consistency. Complications were minimal with hallux varus being the most serious complication with an incidence of 1.5% in their series. Overall patient satisfaction was high.

Goel and Vogel [22] retrospectively reviewed 35 feet that had an offset V osteotomy performed with an average follow-up of 3 years. They found that the osteotomy successfully reduced the intermetatarsal angle, proximal articular set angle, and hallux abductus angle while leaving the first metatarsal length and first metatarsal declination angle unchanged. Patient satisfaction was 94% excellent and good with complete relief from pain in 66% of the patients.

Bettenhausen and Cragel [23] compared patients with either bilateral or unilateral offset V osteotomies. Eighteen patients had bilateral procedures, and 19 patients had unilateral procedures. They found patient satisfaction was essentially equal with 94% excellent and good results for both procedures and similar to Goel and Vogel's result [22]. Overall complications were less frequent in bilateral procedures; however, this was not statistically significant.

Zygmunt, Gudas, and Laros [5] reported on the initial 50 patients upon whom the procedure was performed starting in 1983. Of the 50 patients, 39 were available for reevaluation. Results showed that 85% of the patients were completely satisfied in the cosmesis and function of their foot after the Z bunion-ectomy. No patients were dissatisfied with the cosmesis but 3% were dissatis-fied with the function. The surgeon's satisfaction of the procedure was 79% completely satisfied, 12% mostly satisfied, and 9% dissatisfied. Complications seen in the study included two hallux varus, two fractured metatarsals, and two recurrent hallux valgus, which accounted for the 9% dissatisfaction rate of the surgeon. No patients had complaints of painful internal fixation.

Schoen, Zygmunt, and Gudas [17], in 1989, examined long-term patient satisfaction and objective clinical and radiographic examinations of patients who had undergone the Z bunionectomy at the University of Chicago Medical Center. Fifty-six surgeries were performed on 31 patients, with a follow-up range of 5 to 9 years. Patient satisfaction was rated good to excellent by 90% of the patients. Postoperative radiographic findings included intermetatarsal angle—mean, 7.1 degrees; hallux abductus angle—mean, 8.96 degrees; tibial sesamoidal position—mean, 2.8. mean protrusion was −1.64 mm. Radiographic findings consistent with osteonecrosis were noted of one patient, one foot, although the patient was clinically asymptomatic. The objective findings were as follows: dorsiflexion—mean, 60 degrees; plantarflexion—mean, 14 degrees. No patients had pain or crepitus, nor were they tract-bound in their first metatarsophalangeal joint range of motion. In addition, stance dorsiflexion had a mean of 21 degrees, and the purchase power was 88% good to excellent on plantar paper pull-out testing. First-ray motion qualitatively demonstrated 1.5 to 2 times dorsiflexion to plantarflexion. While some patients had elevatus of the first ray, there were no subsecond metatarsal head keratoses noted. The most common complication in the study was radiographic hallux varus in 205 of the patients, in which none of these patients were symptomatic or dissatisfied. A common anecdotal finding in their study was that while patients returned to work and most activities in the early postoperative months, it took about 1 year before they felt that they were back to "normal." They felt that the long-term favorable patient satisfaction scores obtained in their study indicated that the Z bunionectomy was with-standing the test of time.

Dereymaeker [25] in a follow-up study of 102 feet treated with the scarf modification found an average improvement from 58.6 to 90.8 using the AOFAS forefoot scoring system. Results were compared with the modified Keller Lelievre arthroplasty and distal chevron using the absolute index of the AOFAS score and found that the scarf = 86.3, Chevron = 87.9, and Keller Lelievre = 2.5 points.

Day, White, and DeJesus [21] objectively compared the Z osteotomy with the Kalish osteotomy for HAV correction. They found that there was not any appreciable difference in postoperative results. Both osteotomies provided adequate reduction of increased IMA. In their study, the net change in IMA was greater with the Z osteotomy; however, the average preoperative IMA was also greater. The complication rate was slightly greater with the Kalish series (29%) than with the Z osteotomy (20%) with screw irritation being the greatest complication seen in both groups. None of the commonly associated complications with either the Z osteotomy or the Kalish osteotomy were encountered with this study.

Though most articles on these osteotomies have shown positive results, Coetzee [30] in 2003 reported a high complication rate in 20 patients with a scarf (modified Z) bunionectomy. His complications included 35% loss of height, 5% delayed union and infection, 10% proximal fracture, 30% rotational malunion, and 25% early recurrence of deformity. Forty-five percent of his patients were unsatisfied at 1 year and would not recommend the surgery.

Complications

There are many complications that can occur after any surgical procedure, let alone those particular to the shaft osteotomies. Typically, the potential for complication increased based on two factors: (1) failure to observe indications/contraindications and (2) technical error. Downey [18], when analyzing the complications of the Kalish offset V, found that most complications stemmed from a failure to observe the indications for the procedure. The potential complications (see references [1,2,5,7,9,10,17–22,30]) for these procedures are listed in Box 2.

Some of the complications can be potentially avoided. In the following paragraphs, the major complications of this procedure (overcorrection, undercorrection, fracture, and troughing) and how to avoid them are discussed.

Overcorrection should be avoided as hallux varus is the most likely result (Fig. 18). This may result from aggressive lateral displacement of the osteotomy, creating a negative intermetatarsal correction. Overaggressive tightening of the medial capsule and postoperative bandaging may also create a hallux varus deformity. This complication was the most frequent complication seen in Schoen et al's [17] retrospective study of the Z bunionectomy. This complication is usually the result of a technical error. It is essential in the authors' opinion to use

---

Box 2. Potential complications of shaft osteotomies

Loss of rigid fixation or stability
Infection
Joint stiffness/arthrosis
Delayed union/nonunion
Nerve damage
Troughing
Avascular necrosis
Hallux varus (overcorrection)
Recurrence of deformity (undercorrection)
Fracture of osteotomy or stress fracture

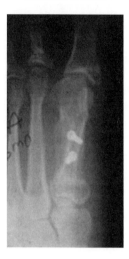

Fig. 18. Hallux varus deformity after osseous overcorrection was performed with a Z osteotomy.

intraoperative imaging before screw placement (Fig. 19) and after capsule closure to ensure that the first ray is in appropriate alignment.

Undercorrection is usually associated with insufficient lateral displacement (Fig. 20). This can be eliminated with repeated loading and imaging of the foot during the surgery after temporary fixation is in place. This potential complication is usually encountered when the procedure is performed on a narrow first metatarsal where the intermetatarsal angle cannot be reduced secondary to limitations of the bone itself or where the intermetatarsal angle is outside the range indicated. Typically, this complication results from a failure to observe indications of an extremely high intermetatarsal angle, where another more proximal procedure should have been performed instead.

Fracture of these osteotomies are most commonly caused by technical error [5,9,18], but can be caused by failure to recognize significant osteopenia or osteoporosis. Fracture of the offset V osteotomy can be caused by either creating

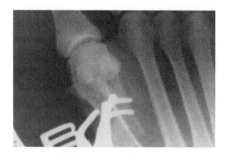

Fig. 19. Intraoperative radiographs may help prevent certain complications that are associated with the Z osteotomy.

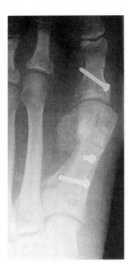

Fig. 20. AP radiograph of an undercorrected Z bunionectomy. Note the recurrence of the deformity radiographically.

too long of a dorsal arm, thereby creating a more acute osteotomy angle, which can cause either an intraarticular fracture at the apex or at the distal spike, or by improper fixation techniques. To avoid fracture caused by the dorsal wing being to long, Downey [18] recommends cutting from proximal to the apex or using an axis guide. Also, if the osteotomy appears to be too long while cutting the bone, the proximal portion of the osteotomy can be notched out vertically to avoid stress at the proximal metatarsal shaft.

Similarly, fracture of Z osteotomy is typically caused by improper osteotomy placement or fixation errors. The reported area of fracture of this osteotomy is at the dorsal cortex at the level of the proximal plantar cut of the osteotomy (Fig. 21). This can be caused by two factors. Either the horizontal cut was not

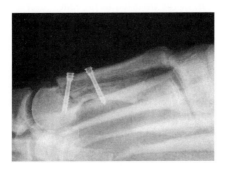

Fig. 21. Lateral radiograph of a fracture of the of the Z osteotomy secondary to improper osteotomy placement and fixation.

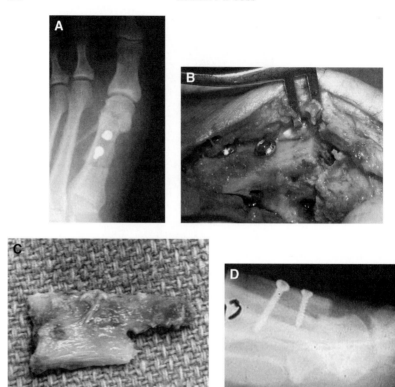

Fig. 22. (*A*) AP radiograph revealing fracture of the plantar wing of the Z osteotomy. (*B, C*) Intraoperative photographs of the patient depicted in the radiograph. Note that there fracture is through the plantar wing and the fracture was caused by the proximal screw not engaging the plantar wing, causing the osteotomy to fail. (*D*) Lateral radiograph of another capital fragment/plantar wing fracture.

two-thirds dorsal and one-third plantar or the proximal plantar cut was beyond the apex of the horizontal wing. Though other authors have advocated the use of the scarf modification or the inverted to prevent this fracture, the authors have found that fracture Z bunionectomy is more likely in the plantar cortex and typically is caused by improper fixation techniques (Fig. 22 and 23). To avoid fractures caused by fixation errors, the surgeon needs to be cognizant of the following: (1) Avoid placement of fixation in the "no-fly zones" (Fig. 16); (2) Avoid placement of fixation too close together. The result can cause a stress riser between the two points of fixation (Fig. 15); (3) Ensure that the fixation has been placed as centrally as possible in both the dorsal and plantar cortices. If the fixation is too close to either the medial or lateral cortices a stress riser can develop; (4) Adequately countersink the screws to prevent stress risers around the screw holes; and (5) Make sure that the fixation penetrates the plantar cortex. If the fixation is within the medullary canal, a cantilever effect can be created, which can fracture the osteotomy when the patient ambulates.

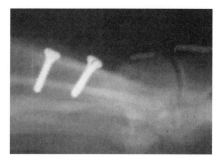

Fig. 23. Example of troughing that occurred when the capital fragment compressed into the medullary canal of the first metatarsal.

Troughing of these osteotomies is also a technical complication, which can lead to elevation of the capital fragment. This in turn can lead to stiffness of the first metatarsophalangeal joint with subsequent arthrosis or possible lateral metatarsalgia and stress fracture. Troughing occurs when the capital fragment compresses into the medullary canal of the first metatarsal, because of poor cortical bone to bone contact between at the osteotomy interface (Fig. 24). Troughing can be typically avoided if the osteotomies are performed correctly and if it occurs to take steps to prevent the osteotomy to be troughed after fixation. To avoid troughing, it is essential when transposing the capital fragment to evaluate whether the medial and lateral cortices will contact the opposite cortex. If this cannot be evaluated, apply the bone reduction forceps with gentle pressure; if the metatarsal head is shifted superiorly, then the cortices may not be contacting and troughing can occur. Troughing can be corrected by two means— swiveling the proximal portion of the osteotomy more laterally or placing bone graft from the medial eminence or overhang into the osteotomy (Fig. 24) to prevent the sinking of the bone into the medullary canal.

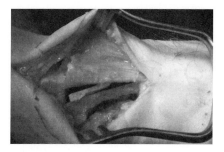

Fig. 24. Troughing can be corrected by placing bone graft from the medial eminence to prevent the sinking of the bone into the meduallary canal.

Summary

Because of its versatility, inherent stability, minimal first metatarsal shortening, good intermetatarsal reduction, and ease of rigid internal fixation, shaft osteotomies are gaining popularity as procedures for the correction of hallux valgus. Strong and stable internal fixation allows for earlier functional recovery and primary bone healing. Several long-term studies have confirmed the surgical reliability of these procedures as a primary procedure for hallux valgus correction (see references [2,5,10,13–15,17,19–23,25]). However, when compared with capital fragment osteotomies of the first metatarsal, shaft osteotomies are slightly more technically demanding, require more dissection, and have a higher surgical learning curve. Complications can be avoided if the surgeon adheres to the indications and technical pitfalls. In closing, shaft osteotomies can provide predictable and rewarding results for the patient and surgeon for the correction of hallux valgus.

References

[1] Vogler H. Shaft osteotomy in hallux valgus reduction. Clin Pod Med 1989;6:47–69.
[2] Kalish SR, Spector JE. The Kalish osteotomy. A review and retrospective analysis of 265 cases. J Am Podiatr Med Assoc 1994;84:237–42.
[3] Meyer M. Eine neue Modifikation der hallux valgus operation. Zbl Chir 1926;53:3265–8.
[4] Burutaran J. Hallux valgus y cortedad anatomica del primer metatarsano (correction quirugica). Actual Med Chir Pied 1976;XIII:261–6.
[5] Zygmunt K, Gudas C, Laros G. Z-bunionectomy with internal screw fixation. J Am Podiatr Med Assoc 1989;79:322–9.
[6] Jarde O, Trinquier-Lautard J, Gabrion A, et al. Hallux valgus treated by first metatarsal scarf osteotomy. A series of 50 cases with a minimum follow up of two years. Rev Chir Orthop Reparatrice App Mot 1999;85:374–80.
[7] Borrelli A, Weil L. Modified scarf bunionectomy: our experience in more than one thousand cases. J Foot Surg 1991;30:609–12.
[8] Glickman S, Zahari D. Short "Z" bunionectomy. J Foot Surg 1986;25:304–6.
[9] Miller J, Stuck R, Sartori M, et al. The inverted Z-bunionectomy: quantitative analysis of the scarf and inverted scarf bunionectomy osteotomies in fresh cadaveric matched pair specimens. J Foot Ankle Surg 1994;33:455–62.
[10] Barouk L. Scarf osteotomy for hallux valgus correction. Local anatomy, surgical technique, and combination with other forefoot procedures. Foot Ankle Clin 2000;5:525–58.
[11] Maestro M, Augoyard M, Barouk LS. Biomecaniques et repere radiologiques du sesamoide lateral de l'hallux par rapport a la palette metatarsienne. Med Chor Pied 1995;11:145–54.
[12] Weil L. Scarf osteotomy for correction of hallux valgus. Historical perspective, surgical technique, and results. Foot Ankle Clin 2000;5:559–80.
[13] Friend G, Grace K, Stone H. Cortical screws versus absorbable pins for fixation of the short Z-bunionectomy. J Foot Ankle Surg 1994;33:411–8.
[14] Kramer J, Barry L, Helfman D, et al. The modified scarf bunionectomy. J Foot Surg 1992; 31:360–7.
[15] Schwartz N, Groves E. Long-term follow-up of internal threaded Kirschner-wire fixation of the scarf bunionectomy. J Foot Surg 1987;26:313–6.
[16] Chang T, Yu G, Ruch J, editors. The inverted scarf bunionectomy. Update 1992: reconstructive surgery of the foot and leg. Tucker (GA): Podiatry Institute Publishing Company; 1992.

[17] Schoen N, Zygmunt K, Gudas C. Z-bunionectomy: retrospective long-term study. J Foot Ankle Surg 1996;35:312–7.

[18] Downey MS. Complications of the Kalish bunionectomy. J Am Podiatr Med Assoc 1994;84: 243–9.

[19] Fox IM, Cuttic M, DeMarco P. The offset V modification of the Chevron bunionectomy: a retrospective study. J Foot Surg 1992;31:615–20.

[20] Kissel CG, Unroe BJ, Parker RM. The offset "V" bunionectomy using cortical screw and buried Kirschner wire fixation. J Foot Surg 1992;31:560–77.

[21] Day R, White S, DeJesus J. The "Z" osteotomy versus the Kalish osteotomy for the correction of hallux abducto valgus deformities: a retrospective analysis. J Foot Ankle Surg 1997; 36:44–50.

[22] Goel R, Vogel B. The offset V osteotomy with screw fixation for correction of hallux valgus: a retrospective study. J Foot Ankle Surg 1993;32:305–10.

[23] Bettenhausen D, Cragel M. The offset-V osteotomy with screw fixation: a retrospective evaluation of unilateral versus bilateral surgery. J Foot Ankle Surg 1997;36:418–21.

[24] Reed T. Allofix freeze-dried cortical bone pins as an alternative to synthetic absorbable polymeric pins: a preliminary study in short Z bunionectomies. J Foot Ankle Surg 1999;38:14–23.

[25] Dereymaker G. Scarf osteotomy for correction of hallux valgus: surgical technique as compared to distal chevron osteotomy. Foot Ankle Clin 2000;5:513–24.

[26] Jacobson K, Gough A, Mendicino SS, Rockett MS. Mechanical comparison of fixation techniques for the offset V osteotomy: a sawbone study. J Foot Ankle Surg 2003;42:339–43.

[27] Khuir J, Wertheimer S, Krueger J, Haut R. Fixation of the offset V osteotomy: mechanical testing of four constructs. J Foot Ankle Surg 2003;42:63–8.

[28] Dalton S, Bauer G, Lamm B, et al. Stability of the offset V osteotomy: effects of fixation, orientation, and surgical translocation in polyurethane foam models and preserved cadaveric specimens. J Foot Ankle Surg 2003;42:53–62.

[29] Popoff I, Negrine JP, Zecovic M, et al. The effect of screw type on the biomechanical properties of scarf and crescentic osteotomies of the first metatarsal. J Foot Ankle Surg 2003;42: 161–4.

[30] Coetzee C. Scarf osteotomy for hallux valgus repair: the dark side. Foot Ankle Int 2003;24: 29–33.

CLINICS IN
PODIATRIC
MEDICINE AND
SURGERY

ELSEVIER
SAUNDERS

Clin Podiatr Med Surg
22 (2005) 197–222

Central Metatarsal Head-Neck Osteotomies: Indications and Operative Techniques

Thomas S. Roukis, DPM

Weil Foot and Ankle Institute, 1455 East Golf Road, Suite 110, Des Plaines, IL 60016, USA

Pathology of the central metatarsals is complicated and involves various potential etiologies [1–8], including (1) soft-tissue pathology (crossover second-toe deformity, plantar plate dyscrasia, skin-related keratotic disorders); (2) structural metatarsal deformities (elongated, plantar displaced, elevated, foreshortened, enlarged plantar condyle(s), posttraumatic malalignment); (3) functional metatarsal deformities (sagittal plane adjacent metatarsal instability or hypermobility, retrograde buckling from associated hammer-toe contractures); and (4) intraarticular pathology (Freiberg's infraction, posttraumatic degenerative joint disease, connective tissue disease, crystalline arthridities). For each of these disorders, there are a host of specific signs and symptoms as well as conservative and surgical treatment options [1–8]. This article focuses specifically on structural metatarsal deformities with some brief discussion regarding soft tissue pathology and functional metatarsal deformities as indicated.

Structural metatarsal deformities include an elongated, plantar-displaced, foreshortened, or elevated metatarsal as well as an enlarged plantar metatarsal head condyle [2]. An elongated, plantar-displaced, or enlarged plantar metatarsal head condyle will create pathology through repeated, concentrated increases in pressure and time (increased force) to the involved central metatarsal [2]. In the "normal" foot, the greatest strain and weight-bearing pressure involves the second metatarsal [9,10]. If the second metatarsal is elongated, plantar displaced, or has an enlarged plantar metatarsal head condyle, these already high strains and pressures could create significant potential for pathology about the metatarsal shaft (stress-fracture) or metatarsal-phalangeal joint (crossover toe deformity, plantar plate dyscrasia, or Freiberg's infraction) [2,9,10]. A foreshortened and

---

E-mail address: troukis@footankledeformity.com

elevated metatarsal will create pathology through increase pressure and time (increased force) to the adjacent metatarsals [2,9,10].

Conservative treatment options have been shown to be successful in alleviating the symptoms associated with structural metatarsal deformities and associated soft tissue pathology and functional metatarsal deformities (see references [1,2,9,11–13]. Conservative treatment options (NSAIDs, ice, topical liniment, intraarticular local anesthetic and corticosteroid injection, and padding and strapping) attempt to reduce any associated synovitis or soft tissue inflammation, accommodate the structural or functional deformity present (ready-made or custom foot orthoses with or without supportive or relieve padding, rocker-sole or stiff-sole shoe gear, cast immobilization, and padding and strapping), or both [2]. Few of these modalities have been studied in depth beyond the use of padding, ready-made insoles, custom foot orthoses, and shoe-gear modifications (see references [2,9,11–13]).

Holmes and Timmerman [9], in a pedobarographic study of five men and five women treated with soft metatarsal pads described a 12% to 60% reduction in plantar pressure for the women and 14% to 40% reduction for the men. Chang et al [11], using an in-shoe pressure sensor system on 10 men treated with soft insoles with metatarsal pads and extradepth shoe gear, determined a statistically significant decrease in pressure-time integrals to the first through fourth metatarsals; a decrease in contact duration to all metatarsal heads; and and increase in peak pressures, contact durations, and pressure-time integrals at the metatarsal shaft region, indicating proximal transfer of weight-bearing forces away from the symptomatic metatarsal head level. Poon and Love [12], using an in-shoe pressure sensor system in 14 patients with metatarsalgia treated with custom foot orthoses with a metatarsal dome (pad), determined a 13% reduction in plantar forefoot pressure and a 71% reduction in pain as determined by an 11-point visual analog pain scale. Finally, Postema et al [13], using a pressure gait analysis system in 42 patients with metatarsalgia treated with custom foot orthoses with a metatarsal pad or a rocker-bar-added extradepth shoe gear, determined a mean reduction in peak plantar forefoot pressure of 15% for the rocker-bar-added extradepth shoe gear and 18% for the custom orthoses with a metatarsal pad.

Despite the paucity of peer-reviewed publications detailing the benefit conservative measures have in the treatment of central metatarsal deformities, they should be attempted for a reasonable period of time before considering surgical intervention. The author's institute has found the use of the previously mentioned conservative modalities to be beneficial in providing sustained and substantial relief of pain in more than 85% of patients being treated for central metatarsal deformities regardless of etiology.

Radiographic analysis

Radiographic analysis is the gold standard by which the metatarsal length pattern or parabola is determined. However, although much has been written about the length pattern between the first and second metatarsals [14–18], little has been written to establish what exactly a "normal" global metatarsal length pattern or parabola should consist of [19–22]. Bojsen-Møller [19] conducted a mechanical study and determined that the most mechanically effective metatarsal length pattern is where the second metatarsal is the longest, the third is the same length as the first, the fourth is shorter than the third, and the fifth is shorter than the fourth (2 > 1 = 3 > 4 > 5). Data from studies involving surgical correction of hallux valgus and hallux rigidus consider the proper relationship between the first and second metatarsals to be when the second metatarsal is ±2 mm longer than the first [14–18]. This data appears to support the findings of Bojsen-Møller [19] in regard to the relationship between the first and second metatarsals but does not further our understanding of the normal length pattern for the remaining lesser metatarsals. More recently, Maestro et al [20] devised a series of complicated measurements to determine the "relative metatarsal length parabola." Maestro et al defined the normal relative metatarsal length parabola according to the "Maestro line" (line passing from the center of the fibular sesamoid, perpendicular to the longitudinal bisection of the second metatarsal, and through the fourth metatarsal head). According to Maestro et al [20] and Barouk [21], after forefoot reconstruction, if the Maestro line does not pass directly through the fourth metatarsal head then further surgical intervention should be employed to accomplish this goal. Maestro et al, in a series of 40 "normal" feet, employed the Maestro line to determine the ideal relative metatarsal length parabola to be when the first metatarsal is equal or 2 mm shorter than the second metatarsal, the third metatarsal is 4 mm (3.4 ± 0.9 mm) shorter than the second, the fourth metatarsal is 6 mm (6.5 ± 1.0 mm) shorter than the third metatarsal, and the fifth metatarsal is 12 mm (12.0 ± 1.9 mm) shorter than the fourth metatarsal (1 = 2 > 3 > 4 > 5 or 1 < 2 > 3 > 4 > 5) [22]. Unfortunately, the techniques employed vary greatly from one study to the next, making any true comparison between the study data and ultimately an established "ideal" or "normal" relative metatarsal length parabola impossible. However, based on the literature available, the ideal relative metatarsal length pattern appears to be when the first and second metatarsals are equal in length and a gentle taper exists between the remaining metatarsals (1 = 2 > 3 > 4 > 5). Proper metatarsal relationships involve the relative length of the metatarsals and the sagittal plane relationship, which should consist of each metatarsal oriented parallel to one another on the weight-bearing surface during the stance and propulsive phases of the gait cycle [2,14,21].

Central metatarsal vascular anatomy

The vascular supply to the central metatarsals has been well established in several anatomic studies [23–25]. The arcuate artery, arising from the dorsalis pedis artery, sends dorsal metatarsal arteries through the intermetatarsal spaces

over the dorsal interosseous muscles that produce a well-defined dorsal capsular network to each of the metatarsal-phalangeal joints. The dorsal capsular
branches anastomose with each other and with the plantar capsular vessels to
form a dense periarticular network that produces one to two fine vessels that
supply the metatarsal head at the level of the extraarticular dorsal synovial fold
and collateral ligament attachments. The plantar arch, arising from the lateral
plantar artery division of the posterior tibial artery, sends plantar metatarsal
arteries through the intermetatarsal spaces between the plantar interosseous
muscles and the oblique head of the adductor hallucis muscle. These vessels
produce a well-defined and robust (0.5–0.8 mm) branch that divides into two
clearly defined terminal branches at the level of the plantar metatarsal metaphyseal-diaphyseal junction ("axilla" or "cul-de-sac") and proximal attachment
of the plantar plate. One branch supplies the plantar capsular structures
including the plantar plate and anastomoses with the dorsal capsular branches
and the other supplies the metatarsal head itself [23–25]. The nutrient artery
and periosteal vessels are also important and supply the metaphyseal and
cortical components of the metatarsal, respectively [23,25]. However, because
this article focuses on central metatarsal head-neck osteotomies, any osteotomy
at this level should limit soft tissue dissection through the interspaces, about
the capsule and periosteal structures, and spare the plantar metaphyseal-diaphyseal junction.

Central metatarsal osteotomies

Since Meisenbach's [26] description of a midshaft central metatarsal
osteotomy in 1916, more than 40 procedures and modifications have been
described in the literature [27–34]. These procedures include (1) partial or total
plantar condylectomy, metatarsal head resection, and ray resection; (2) metatarsal head-neck shortening, dorsiflexory, peg-in-hole, and combined osteotomies;
(3) midshaft shortening and dorsiflexory metatarsal osteotomies; and (4) base
shortening and dorsiflexory metatarsal osteotomies [26–34]. Despite the plethora
of central metatarsal osteotomies described, issues such as the optimum type of
osteotomy, level of osteotomy, role and type of fixation employed, necessity
and duration of restricted weight bearing, and the role of performing multiple
central metatarsal osteotomies remain poorly defined.

The author discusses three specific central metatarsal head-neck osteotomies
and their modifications: (1) the minimal incision or percutaneous osteotomy [28];
(2) the Weil metatarsal osteotomy [33,35–44]; and (3) the "telescoping"
osteotomy. These specific osteotomies were chosen based on their unique appli-
cations, popularity or lack thereof, and novelty. The head-neck level was chosen
because this is the level at which most recent publications discussing central
metatarsal osteotomies have focused and is the one most widely chosen by
practicing foot and ankle surgeons.

Minimal incision (percutaneous) osteotomy

Minimal incision or percutaneous osteotomy of the central metatarsals has received little attention in the literature [28]; however, this a valuable procedure for treating multiple central metatarsal deformities following iatrogenic injury, trauma with malunion, or plantar diabetic neuropathic ulcerations recalcitrant to healing or recurrent despite appropriate conservative measures (Lowell Scott Weil, Sr., DPM, personal communication, 2001).

The surgical technique begins with the patient positioned in the supine position on the operating room table. The use of an ankle tourniquet is optional and not routinely employed because of the limited soft tissue dissection afforded by this procedure. Following either local anesthesia alone or combined with intravenous sedation, a 1-cm transverse incision is placed through the skin at the dorsal aspect of the appropriate metatarsal surgical neck and dissected down to the level of the capsule and periosteum using a hemostat with the jaws fully closed. Once the bone is directly palpated, the hemostat jaws are opened with one jaw placed medially and the other laterally until the hemostat can be advanced from dorsal to plantar. This elevates the soft tissue from the medial, dorsal, and lateral aspects of the metatarsal surgical neck. Under direct image intensification, a power saw is used to create an osteotomy from dorsal to plantar and slightly biased from proximal to distal to allow for dorsal and proximal translation of the capital fragment. Alternatively, a predictable maneuver the author has used to identify the proper osteotomy level is to place the thumb of the nondominant hand directly over the metatarsal head or plantar keratotic lesion. The index finger of the nondominant hand is then placed over the dorsal aspect of the metatarsal in line with the thumb. This creates an "okay" sign and identifies the proximal extent of the metatarsal surgical neck where the osteotomy should be performed (Lowell Scott Weil, Sr., DPM, personal communication, 2001).

Following completion of the osteotomy, a small osteotome is inserted to verify completion of the osteotomy. Percutaneous Kirschner wire or breakaway-type pins can be used to stabilize the osteotomy but are usually not necessary as the intention is for the capital fragment to "seek its own level" rather than be rigidly fixated. The surgical site is irrigated and the skin is closed with a single absorbable suture. A light dressing is applied with extra padding directly underneath the capital fragment to maintain dorsal translation and the patient is placed directly back into an athletic shoe or roomy oxford with full weight bearing to tolerance allowed. The initial surgical dressings are removed in 7 to 10 days and the patient placed back into regular shoe gear as tolerated.

White [28], in a limited retrospective review of 62 second metatarsal, 29 third metatarsal, and 17 fourth metatarsal minimal incision unfixated osteotomies, found two delayed unions (0.3%), one (2%) malunion, and no nonunions all for the second metatarsal [28]. The delayed unions were attributed to improper placement of the osteotomy distal to the metaphyseal-diaphyseal junction (metatarsal head-neck junction), thereby disrupting the vascular supply to the capitol fragment as previously discussed. Because of the paucity of peer-reviewed published literature, the routine use of minimal incision osteotomies about the central metatarsals should be performed with caution.

Weil metatarsal osteotomy

The Weil metatarsal osteotomy has received much attention in the medical literature regarding central metatarsal abnormalities (metatarsalgia, intractable plantar keratotic lesions, crossover second-toe deformity, length abnormalities, rheumatoid joint salvage, medial, and lateral lesser digit angulation at the metatarsal-phalangeal joint level) [33,35–45] and has even been applied to the hand for metacarpal deformities [46]. The Weil metatarsal osteotomy involves minimal soft tissue dissection, is easy to perform, allows precise placement of the plantar capitol fragment, can involve multiple modifications, is inherently stable in design requiring a minimal amount of internal fixation, and allows for immediate guarded weight bearing [33,35].

The surgical technique for either osteotomy begins with the patient positioned in the supine position on the operating room table. Following local anesthesia alone or combined with intravenous sedation, the foot and ankle is exsanguinated with an elastic bandage and an ankle tourniquet inflated for hemostasis. A dorsal, curvilinear incision extending from the distal one quarter of the lesser metatarsal to the proximal interphalangeal joint of the associated digit is performed if a concomitant digital procedure is to be performed. In the rare instance that only the Weil metatarsal osteotomy is to be performed, a small "smile" incision placed at the level of the lesser metatarsal surgical neck can be used and will afford enough exposure to perform the osteotomy and place internal fixation [35]. Regardless, the incision is deepened directly through the skin, superficial fascia, and adipose to the level of the capsule and periosteum overlying the lesser metatarsal-phalangeal joint. Several approaches to the lesser metatarsal-phalangeal joint are possible and include (1) splitting the natural junction between the extensor digitorum longus and brevis (no transverse plane digit deviation); (2) direct medial incision (lateral digit deviation); and (3) direct lateral incision (medial digit deviation) depending on the presence or absence of an angular deformity to the digit at the lesser metatarsal-phalangeal joint level [33,35]. Once the extensor tendon complex has been incised the capsule and periosteum is then reflected using a surgical scalpel and periosteal elevator to expose the dorsal, medial, and lateral aspects of the lesser metatarsal head and neck. The osteotomy begins at a level 2 mm below the dorsal articular cartilage of the lesser metatarsal head and is angled proximally is such a manner as to extend to the junction of the distal and middle one third of the metatarsal (just proximal to the plantar metaphyseal-diaphyseal junction termed the axilla or cul-de-sac of the lesser metatarsal) [33,35]. This angle approximates a 10° to 15° plantar angle compared with the longitudinal axis of the metatarsal which in turn is plantar declinated in relation to the weight-bearing surface of the foot [33,35]. A "pure" Weil osteotomy is performed by completing the osteotomy through the plantar diaphysis creating two separate osseous segments. The plantar capitol fragment will readily migrate proximally and almost always "settles" at the desired level of shortening. However, this should be verified with intraoperative image intensification or through the placement of sterile small-gauge needles inserted into the adjacent metatarsal-phalangeal joints to properly determine the appropriate degree of shortening to balance the metatarsal parabola as previously described. If more than 3 mm of shortening is performed for any of the central metatarsals, a small "slice" of bone must be removed form the plantar capitol fragment as it has a larger bone mass than the remaining metatarsal shaft [33,47]. Because the osteotomy is performed at an angle other than horizontal (directed 10–15° plantarly), the capitol fragment will migrate plantarly and proximally and can create a new symptomatic proximal plantar prominence if left uncorrected (see references [33,42,44,47]). The plantar capital fragment is then held in full apposition with either a small scoop-type elevator or with the index finger from the surgeon's nondominant hand providing dorsally directed pressure at the proximal extent of the osteotomy and fixated with one or two small-diameter nonlag screws (Fig. 1). The use of provisional Kirschner wire fixation and specialized bone clamps can also be used to maintain position, but the author has found these techniques cumbersome and unnecessary for routine use. Any redundant dorsal osseous prominence is then gently resected with a Rongeur to a normal anatomical configuration.

Several modifications to the Weil metatarsal osteotomy exist and include (1) tilt up; (2) tilt down; (3) medial transposition; and (4) lateral transposition of the plantar capitol fragment (see references [33,40,44,48]).

The tilt-up Weil metatarsal osteotomy is indicated in the presence of a prominent plantar condyle and resultant intractable plantar keratoma with an appropriate metatarsal length pattern or in the presence of degenerative joint changes (Freiberg's infraction) [33,44]. The tilt-up Weil metatarsal osteotomy is performed as described except that the plantar-proximal cortical-periosteal junction is gently "feathered" in such a fashion as to allow motion between the dorsal and plantar capitol fragments but not result in two separate fragments. A small (1–2 mm) wedge of bone is then resected from the plantar capital fragment, as this has a larger bone volume than does the remaining metatarsal neck and shaft. The plantar capital fragment is then tilted in a dorsal direction, held in full apposition and fixated with one or two small-diameter nonlag screws. Any redundant dorsal osseous prominence is then gently resected with a Rongeur.

The tilt-down Weil metatarsal osteotomy is a fairly new modification intended to limit the tendency for postoperative dorsal contracture of the lesser digit (extensus contracture) [33]. The tilt-down Weil metatarsal osteotomy is essentially an inverted tilt-up osteotomy. Specifically, a small (1–2 mm) proximally based wedge of bone is resected from the remaining metatarsal shaft rather than the plantar capitol fragment, as the wedge removed is proximally based and the remaining metatarsal shaft has a greater volume of bone. The plantar capital fragment is then tilted in a plantar direction, held in full apposition as described previously, and fixated with one or two small-diameter nonlag

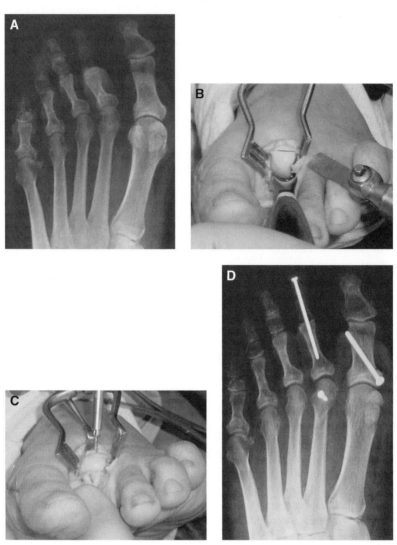

Fig. 1. Anterior-posterior radiograph demonstrating an elongated second metatarsal relative to the adjacent first and third metatarsals. The patient had symptomatic second metatarsal-phalangeal joint plantar metatarsal head pain, symptomatic hallux valgus, and second hammer digit syndrome (*A*). Intraoperative photograph demonstrating the proper Weil osteotomy level (2 mm intraarticular from the dorsal articular cartilage) and the use of a scoop-type elevator to maintain reduction of the osteotomy (*B*) followed by rigid internal fixation with a small-diameter cortical screw (*C*). The screw lengths typically vary between 10 mm and 14 mm. Postoperative radiograph demonstrating the properly fixated Weil metatarsal osteotomy as well as intramedullary screw fixation of the second digit and a modified McBride bunionectomy with Akin great toe osteotomy (*D*).

screws. Any redundant dorsal osseous prominence is then gently resected with a Rongeur.

The medial transposition Weil metatarsal osteotomy modification is indicated in the presence of a medially deviated or crossover second-toe deformity [33,40,48]. The medial transposition Weil metatarsal osteotomy is performed as described previously except that the plantar capitol fragment is transposed in a medial direction one third to one half the width of the remaining metatarsal shaft. By medially transposing the plantar capitol fragment, the digit will assume a more lateral position similar to the effect lateral transposition of the first metatarsal head has on the reduction of the hallux abductus angle and balancing of the first metatarsal-phalangeal joint [33]. The plantar capital fragment is then held in full apposition as described and fixated with one or two small-diameter nonlag screws. Any redundant dorsal osseous prominence is then gently resected with a Rongeur.

The lateral transposition Weil metatarsal osteotomy modification is indicated in the presence of a laterally deviated digit (rheumatoid lesser metatarsal-phalangeal joint deformity) [33,40]. The lateral transposition Weil metatarsal osteotomy is performed as described except that the plantar capitol fragment is transposed in a lateral direction one third to one half the width of the remaining metatarsal shaft. By laterally transposing the plantar capitol fragment, the digit will assume a more medial position for the reasons described previously. The plantar capital fragment is then held in full apposition and fixated with one or two small-diameter nonlag screws. Any redundant dorsal osseous prominence is then gently resected with a Rongeur.

Following irrigation of the surgical site, the associated lesser digit is held in an overcorrected plantarflexed position, and the extensor tendon complex is repaired with heavy-gauge absorbable sutures. The remaining deep tissues and skin edges are reapproximated using the surgeon's preferred technique, although a running subcuticular suture and adhesive bandage application will allow earlier bathing and negate the need to remove sutures at a later date.

All of the Weil metatarsal osteotomy modifications allow for immediate weight bearing in a bulky, well-padded surgical dressing and postoperative shoe. Because the sutures are absorbable, the patient is allowed to bathe and shower after the initial dressings are removed and instructed to leave the adhesive dressings alone until they come off with wear. A sling-type toe brace is employed for the first 6 to 8 weeks to maintain the digit in a plantarflexed posture and limit the potential for secondary dorsal scar tissue induced migration of the digit (floating toe syndrome) (Fig. 2). Additionally, the patient is instructed to per-form active and passive plantarflexion home physical therapy multiple times throughout the day to further prevent a dorsiflexion or extensus contracture as well as strengthen the intrinsic musculature and flexor apparatus for long-term digit stabilization. Because the Weil metatarsal osteotomy is inherently stable, the patient is initially placed into a gym shoe or roomy oxford to limit postoperative edema; once this subsides, the patient is allowed to return to regular shoe gear [33]. The patient is allowed to return to activities as soon as pain subsides, and

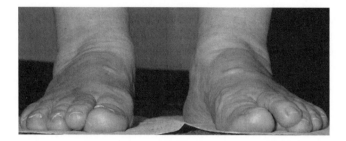

Fig. 2. Postoperative photograph following a Weil metatarsal osteotomy of the second metatarsal bilateral. The right foot (left side of picture) also had a flexor tendon transfer performed, whereas the left foot (right side of picture) had only an isolated Weil metatarsal osteotomy. Notice the persistent static elevation of the second digit on the left foot, which is a frequent complication of the Weil metatarsal osteotomy performed in isolation.

should be seen at regular intervals to assess the incision site healing and any other related issues.

Although no formal publications are available in the medical literature, Lowell Scott Weil, Sr., DPM, initially performed this procedure in 1985 and shared this technique with L. Samuel Barouk, MD during a meeting in France in 1992 [33]. Since that time, much has been written about the Weil metatarsal osteotomy and its modifications, exclusively in the orthopedic literature [35–45].

Rochwerger et al [36] performed a comparison of the Weil metatarsal osteotomy (N = 56 feet) with a base osteotomy and soft tissue rebalancing of the metatarsal-phalangeal joint (N = 75 feet) in isolated second metatarsal pathology (19 instabilities, 43 subluxations, 69 dislocations). These authors determined that the Weil metatarsal osteotomy was better suited to correct the relative length abnormality of the second metatarsal, and this correlated with significantly improved results (less deformity recurrence, less transfer metatarsalgia, and less pain with ambulation) [36]. Maceira et al [37], in a review of 403 Weil metatarsal osteotomies performed for "first ray insufficiency syndromes and related deformities," determined that shortening of greater than 5 mm in the second metatarsal and greater than 6 mm in the third metatarsal predisposed the lesser metatarsal-phalangeal joint to develop postoperative stiffness. Mühlbauer et al [38] performed a retrospective clinical and radiographic analysis of the Weil metatarsal osteotomy in 30 patients (69 osteotomies) with various metatarsal-phalangeal joint pathology (relative length abnormality, plantar keratotic formation, or joint subluxation). The mean shortening achieved was 4.4 mm. Subluxation of the lesser metatarsal-phalangeal joint was corrected in 18 of 22 patients (81%). Although satisfaction was high, restricted plantarflexion of the metatarsal-phalangeal joint was a common problem (16 patients; 73%), and the authors advocated early postoperative physical therapy to minimize this complication [38].

Trnka et al [39] performed a retrospective review of 30 patients (47 metatarsals) treated with either a Weil metatarsal osteotomy (N = 25) or Helal osteotomy (oblique dorsal-proximal sliding distal-shaft osteotomy) (N = 22) followed for a mean of 22 months. The mean shortening was 4.4 mm for the Weil metatarsal osteotomy group. The patients managed with the Weil metatarsal osteotomy had significantly higher satisfaction, lower incidence of recurrent metatarsalgia (0% versus 27%), fewer transfer lesions (0% versus 41%), and a higher percentage of radiographic reduction and maintenance of lesser metatarsal-phalangeal joint dislocation (84% versus 36%). There were no malunions or pseudoarthroses appreciated in the Weil metatarsal osteotomy group compared with five malunions and three pseudoarthroses in the Helal osteotomy group [39]. Davies and Saxby [40] reviewed 47 Weil metatarsal osteotomies for various metatarsal-phalangeal joint pathology (relative length abnormalities, hallux valgus with plantar second metatarsal-phalangeal joint pathology, lesser metatarsal-phalangeal joint instability, and malunion). The mean shortening was 4.1 mm. Transfer lesions developed in one (2%) patient, and recurrent metatarsal-phalangeal joint subluxation occurred in one (2%) patient with no instances of avascular necrosis. Restricted plantarflexion of the metatarsal-phalangeal joint was a common finding but "with aggressive physical therapy it was not a problem at final follow-up," which was at a mean of 9 months [40].

Vandeputte et al [41] performed a clinical and pedobarographic analysis of 59 Weil metatarsal osteotomies for either plantar keratotic lesions or dislocated metatarsal-phalangeal joints with a mean follow-up of 30 months. The mean shortening was 5.9 mm. Complete resolution of the plantar keratotic lesions occurred in 44 patients (75%), and partial resolution occurred in 12 (20%). Two incidents of transfer plantar keratotic lesions occurred and recurrent dislocations occurred in five joints (15%). Comparison of the pre- and postoperative pedobarographic measurements showed a significant decreased load under the affected metatarsal head. There were no nonunions or malunions appreciated. Although total lesser metatarsal-phalangeal joint range of motion was universally diminished, plantar toe purchase was maintained [41]. Trnka et al [42] performed a cadaveric and three-dimensional sawbone model study to determine the potential cause of lesser metatarsal-phalangeal joint stiffness following a Weil metatarsal osteotomy to the second metatarsal. The sawbone portion of the study compared the degree of shortening with the degree of plantar depression of the capitol fragment for various angles of the Weil metatarsal osteotomy relative to the long-axis of the metatarsal. The authors were unable to achieve an osteotomy angle less than 25° as the saw blade deflected off of the second metatarsal cortex in each attempt. Because the second metatarsal is considered to be 15° declinated relative to the weight-bearing surface, and no osteotomy less than 25° could be performed, the plane of the osteotomy was always 10° or greater and resulted in concomitant depression with proximal transposition of the capitol fragment. The mean depression following a 25° osteotomy was 3.03 mm (5.03 mm shortening) and following a 40° osteotomy was 4.2 mm (3.65 mm shortening). The cadaveric portion of the study likewise revealed a consistent plantar depression of the capitol fragment that alters the lesser metatarsal-phalangeal joint center of rotation. The authors believed that this in turn converts the interosseous muscles to function as dorsiflexors rather than plantarflexors as their location is now through or dorsal to the axis of rotation that also allows the extensor tendons to act unopposed and further dorsiflex the digit. The authors recommended lengthening the extensor tendons, provisional transarticular Kirschner wire fixation, flexor tendon transfer, and aggressive postoperative physical therapy as appropriate techniques to employ to prevent postoperative stiffness and dorsiflexion contracture of the lesser metatarsal-phalangeal joint [42].

Tollafield [43] evaluated the Weil metatarsal osteotomy in 47 metatarsals and determined complete resolution of plantar keratotic lesions in five patients (36%), two patients (8%) developed symptomatic transfer lesions, and seven patients (22%) developed symptomatic elevation of the lesser metatarsal-phalangeal joint. The authors recommended lengthening the extensor tendon complex, flexor tendon transfer, postoperative splinting, and aggressive physical therapy to limit the instance of digit elevation and diminished toe purchase, but stated that "no substantial research has been developed to assist this theory." The author further states that "lesser metatarsal surgery is unforgiving" and requires further quality outcomes-driven research [43]. Melamed et al [44] performed a sawbone analysis of 40 Weil metatarsal osteotomies with and without excision of a 5-mm dorsally based wedge of bone or 5-mm slice of bone. All of the osteotomies were performed 30° to the long-axis of the second metatarsal and underwent a 5-mm proximal transposition of the capitol fragment. A mean shortening of 5.3 mm and plantar depression of 2.1 mm occurred in the unmodified Weil metatarsal osteotomy group; a mean shortening of 8.1 mm and plantar depression of 0.8 mm occurred in the dorsally based wedge resection modification group; and a mean shortening of 16.9 mm and plantar depression of 3.3 mm occurred in the 5-mm slice. Mathematical calculations determined that removal of each 1 mm of dorsally based wedge results in 0.5 mm of shortening and 0.6 mm of elevation. The authors concluded that removing a dorsally based wedge of bone can reduce or eliminate unwanted plantar displacement of the capitol fragment and is indicated when excessive shortening or preexisting metatarsalgia contraindicate the use of an unmodified Weil metatarsal osteotomy.

Finally, O'Kane and Kilmartin [45] performed an analysis of 20 Weil metatarsal osteotomies to the second and third metatarsals (17 patients) for treatment of central metatarsalgia with a mean follow-up of 18 months. The mean shortening of the second metatarsal was 5.2 mm, and the mean shortening of the third metatarsal was 5.4 mm. There were no nonunions or malunions appreciated. One patient (6%) developed transfer metatarsalgia to the fourth metatarsal, one patient (6%) had recurrence of their initial symptoms, four patients (24%) developed postoperative stiffness at the lesser metatarsal-phalangeal joints, and eight patients (47%) developed persistent elevation of the digits. The authors concluded that although persistent digit elevation and stiffness are common findings following a Weil metatarsal osteotomy, these findings were not a cause of patient dissatisfaction and their clinical significance has yet to be determined [45].

Despite high patient satisfaction and consistent resolution of painful lesser metatarsal symptomatology and pathology, the Weil metatarsal osteotomy and its modifications are not without potential complications. Careful patient selection, attention to detail regarding the orientation, degree of shortening, and concomitant use of the modifications presented as well as judicial use of ancillary soft tissue procedures and aggressive postoperative physical therapy should be employed to limit the incidence of symptomatic lesser metatarsal-phalangeal joint stiffness and digit elevation following the Weil metatarsal osteotomy.

Telescoping metatarsal osteotomy

The "telescoping" metatarsal osteotomy is a novel procedure and is indicated in the presence of an abnormal central metatarsal length pattern (James B. Ringstrom, DPM, personal communication, 1997) (Fig. 3A). This central metatarsal osteotomy involves minimal soft tissue dissection, is easy to perform, and allows for precise shortening but is inherently unstable and requires a period of protected partial weight bearing to avoid hardware failure and resultant complications.

The surgical technique for either osteotomy begins with the patient positioned in the supine position on the operating room table. Following local anesthesia alone or combined with intravenous sedation, the foot and ankle is exsanguinated with an elastic bandage and an ankle tourniquet inflated for hemostasis. A dorsal, curvilinear incision extending from the distal one third of the lesser metatarsal to the proximal interphalangeal joint of the associated digit is performed if a concomitant digital procedure is to be performed. Otherwise, the incision terminates at the level of the metatarsal-phalangeal joint. Regardless, the incision is deepened directly through the skin, superficial fascia, and adipose to the level of the capsule and periosteum overlying the lesser metatarsal-phalangeal joint. Several approaches to the lesser metatarsal-phalangeal joint are possible as previously described. Once the extensor tendon complex has been incised, the capsule and periosteum is reflected using a surgical scalpel and periosteal elevator to expose the dorsal, medial, and lateral aspects of the lesser metatarsal head, neck, and distal shaft. At a level just proximal to the metaphyseal-diaphyseal junction (surgical neck) a vertical through-and-through osteotomy is performed. A second through-and-through osteotomy is then performed proximal to the first one, the desired amount of shortening to be performed (Fig. 3B) taking into account the "kerf" or bone resected from the width of the saw blade (usually 1 mm for each osteotomy). The resultant cylinder of bone is then removed from the surgical site and the distal capitol fragment transposed proximally to directly appose the remaining metatarsal shaft (Fig. 3C). The osteotomy is fixated with either a large diameter smooth Steinman pin in intramedullary fashion (James B. Ringstrom, DPM, personal communication, 1997) [49] or a condylar plate and screw system (Synthes, Paoli, Pennsylvania) (Fig. 3D). The intramedullary fixation involves sequential reaming of the proximal metatarsal shaft until a "tight" fit is achieved, at which point the pin is cut with approximately 5 to 6 mm extending from the metatarsal shaft. The distal capitol fragment is then impaled onto the exposed pin in "shish-kebab" fashion with care taken to make certain

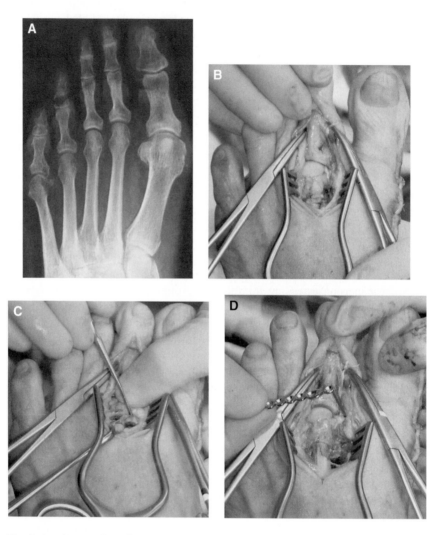

Fig. 3. Anterior-posterior radiograph demonstrating an elongated second metatarsal relative to the adjacent first and third metatarsals. The patient had symptomatic second metatarsal-phalangeal joint plantar metatarsal head pain as well as symptomatic hallux valgus and second hammer digit syndrome (A). Intraoperative photograph demonstrating the level and amount of bone resected for the telescoping metatarsal osteotomy (B). The cylinder of resected bone is shown being removed with the aide of a Freer elevator (C). Photograph of the condylar "blade" plate before cutting the "barb" to proper length for insertion into the metatarsal head fragment (D). Final intraoperative photograph of the condylar plate after insertion of all screws, demonstrating the close osseous apposition achieved through offset drilling of the proximal screw holes (E). Postoperative radiograph demonstrating the properly fixated telescoping metatarsal osteotomy as well as intramedullary screw fixation of the second digit and a modified McBride bunionectomy with Akin great toe osteotomy (F).

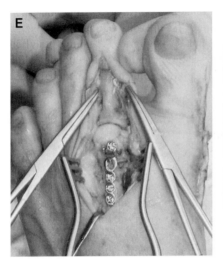
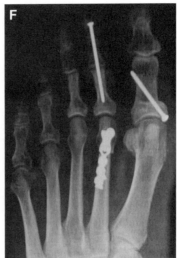

Fig. 3 (*continued*).

the pin does not violate the metatarsal head and enter the metatarsal-phalangeal joint (Fig. 4). The condylar plate and screw fixation involves the use of a 2-mm condylar "blade" plate with the original "barb" cut to a length corresponding to the depth of the metatarsal head (usually 12–14 mm) (Synthes, Paoli, Pennsylvania). A 1.5-mm drill is used to create a hole from dorsal to plantar in the metatarsal head just proximal to the dorsal extent of the articular cartilage into which the condylar plate barb is impaled. The screw hole adjacent to the barb is then filled with the appropriate length screw, thereby securely fixating the distal capitol fragment. Using an offset drilling technique (drill hole placed at the proximal extent of the screw hole closest to the osteotomy), direct linear compression is achieved across the osteotomy site, and the remaining screw holes are sequentially filled (Fig. 3E, F). Following irrigation of the surgical site, the associated lesser digit is held in an overcorrected plantarflexed position and the extensor tendon complex is repaired with heavy gauge absorbable sutures. The remaining deep tissues and skin edges are reapproximated using the surgeons preferred technique, although a running subcuticular suture and adhesive bandage application will allow earlier bathing and negate the need to remove sutures at a later date.

The telescoping central metatarsal osteotomy allows for immediate, partial, or touchdown weight bearing in a bulky, well-padded surgical dressing and post-operative shoe but not unassisted, full weight bearing because of the inherent instability of the osteotomy and reliance on internal fixation alone to afford stability. However, because the sutures are absorbable, the patient is allowed to bathe and shower after the initial dressings are removed and instructed to leave the adhesive dressings alone until they come off with wear. As with the Weil

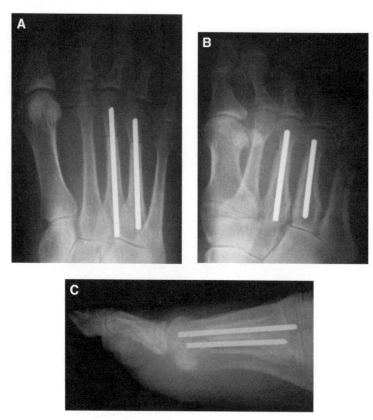

Fig. 4. Postoperative anterior-posterior (*A*), oblique (*B*), and lateral (*C*) radiographs following telescoping osteotomies of the third and fourth metatarsals fixated with intramedullary nail fixation. Note the close osseous apposition achieved with this technique.

metatarsal osteotomy, a sling-type toe brace is employed for the first 6 to 8 weeks to maintain the digit in a plantarflexed posture and limit the potential for secondary dorsal scar tissue induced migration of the digit (floating toe syndrome). Additionally, the patient is instructed to perform active and passive plantarflexion home physical therapy multiple times throughout the day to further prevent a dorsiflexion or extensus contracture and to strengthen the intrinsic musculature and flexor apparatus for long-term digit stabilization. Once serial radiographs and clinical examination reveal osseous healing, the patient is placed into a gym shoe or roomy oxford to limit postoperative edema. Once this subsides the patient is allowed to return to regular shoe gear and normal activities as soon as pain subsides. They should be seen at regular intervals to assess the incision site healing and any other related issues.

No formal published manuscripts are available in the medical literature regarding the telescoping central metatarsal osteotomy described here, and its use remains a matter for conjecture.

Concomitant lesser digit procedures

Lesser digital procedures performed concomitantly with central metatarsal osteotomies involve sagittal or transverse plane deformity correction through the use of a (1) proximal interphalangeal joint arthrodesis [7,8,50]; (2) flexor digitorum longus tendon transfer (see references [5,6,51,52]); (3) extensor digitorum brevis tendon transposition [53]; (4) min-Akin (Akinette) osteotomy of the base of the proximal phalanx [54]; or (5) metallic hemi-implant (resurfacing endoprosthesis).

Arthrodesis of the proximal interphalangeal joint has been well described in the literature [7,8] and can involve the use of temporary Kirschner wire fixation or buried internal fixation [50]. This procedure is used in the presence of a rigid

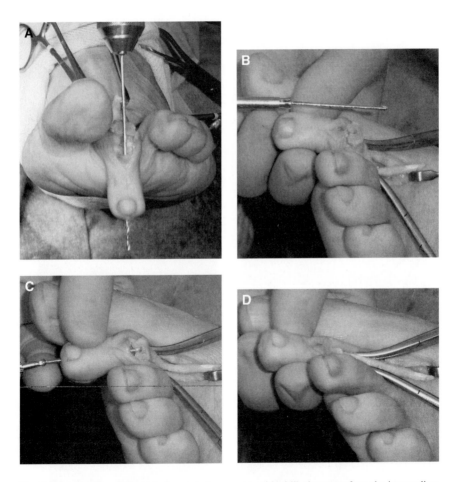

Fig. 5. Intraoperative photograph demonstrating proper guide drill placement from the intermediate phalanx through the distal tip of the second toe (A) followed by insertion of the small-diameter, long screw in intramedullary nail fashion (B–D).

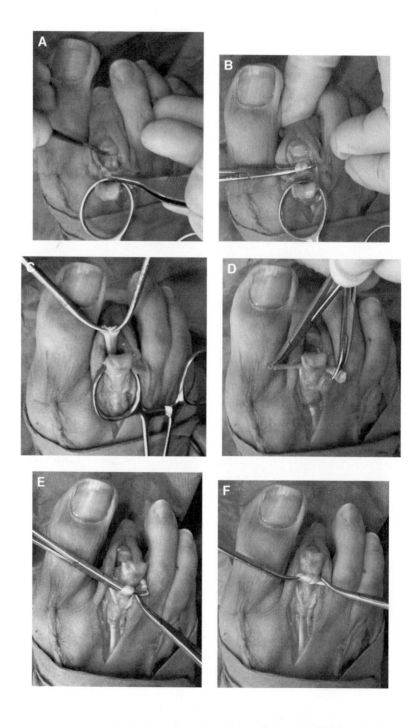

hammer toe contracture or a spastic flexible hammer toe contracture with retrograde buckling and persistent central metatarsal head plantar prominence despite full correction of any length or sagittal plane abnormality following one of the central metatarsal osteotomies described previously. Following preparation of the proximal interphalangeal joint through the surgeons preferred technique (end-to-end, cup-and-cone, or peg-in-hole resection), the author prefers to use a long, small-diameter cortical screw (Synthes, USA, Paoli, Pennsylvania) placed as an intramedullary nail to stabilize the proximal interphalangeal arthrodesis site and the distal interphalangeal joint in slight flexion. This is performed by drilling a guide hole in the exposed proximal phalanx shaft and another guide hole from the base of the intermediate phalanx out the end of the digit distally. A long, small-diameter cortical screw (2 mm diameter, 40 mm length) is then driven from the tip of the digit across the distal and proximal interphalangeal joints (Fig. 5). Because the hardware is internal and buried, this technique has several advantages over previously described external and internal fixation techniques: (1) early bathing is permitted without fear of pin-tract infection; (2) persistent compression and maintenance of reduction is afforded; and (3) it can be rapidly performed in a timely fashion. The only relative disadvantage is that the end result is a rigid digit that is incapable of motion at the distal interphalangeal joint. The author believes this represents no disadvantage at all as the distal interphalangeal joint is slightly flexed at the time of screw insertion, the development of a mallet toe contracture is avoided, and the rigid "beam" effect created afforded by the pull of the flexor tendons negates the need to perform a flexor tendon transfer in all but the most unstable metatarsal-phalangeal joints.

Transfer of the flexor digitorum longus tendon to the dorsal aspect of the base of the proximal phalanx has received much attention in the literature (see references [5,6,51,52]) and is indicated when the digit remains unstable in the sagittal plane following central metatarsal osteotomy. Although the pathologic process involved in sagittal plane instability or frank dislocation primarily involves attenuation or rupture of the plantar plate, primary repair of the plantar plate is not routinely used because of difficult dissection, poor tissue quality, and tendency to create a rigid, nonfunctional metatarsal-phalangeal joint. Instead, transfer of the flexor digitorum longus tendon to the dorsal aspect of the base of the proximal phalanx is the preferred technique. The flexor tendon can be harvested from many different incision techniques and secured through various techniques (simple sutures, drill holes, tendon anchors). However, the author's preferred technique involves a single dorsal incision through which the proximal

---

Fig. 6. Cadaveric dissection specimen demonstrating harvest of the flexor digitorum longus tendon through the proximal interphalangeal joint for transfer. The proximal phalanx is elevated, thereby exposing the plantar plate to the proximal interphalangeal joint, which has been incised to expose the flexor digitorum brevis tendon slips (A). A Hemostat is placed deep between the flexor digitorum brevis tendon slips to capture the flexor digitorum longus tendon (B), which is transected distally and brought into the surgical field (C). The flexor digitorum longus tendon has been split along its central raphe and transferred to the dorsal aspect of the base of the proximal phalanx (D) where it is sequentially tied into a knot and tensioned (E,F).

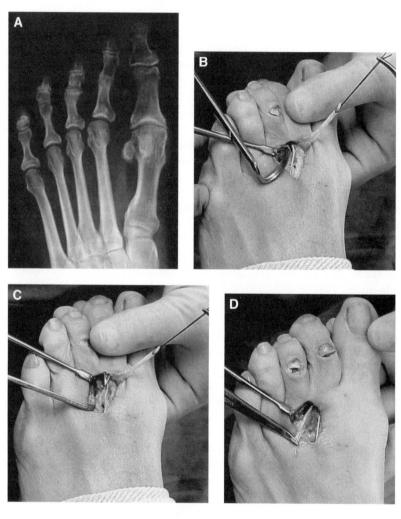

Fig. 7. Anterior-posterior radiograph demonstrating a medially angulated second digit at the metatarsal-phalangeal joint level as well as hammer digit syndrome to the third, fourth, and fifth digits following previous proximal interphalangeal joint arthrodesis to the second digit and modified McBride bunionectomy to the first metatarsal-phalangeal joint (*A*). Intraoperative photograph demonstrating harvest of the extensor digitorum brevis tendon (right side elevated with suture) and a curved "tonsil" wire passer used to transfer the tendon (*B*). The wire passer has been placed from proximal to distal within the second interdigital space deep to the deep transverse intermetatarsal ligament (*C*). The extensor digitorum brevis tendon has been rerouted deep to the deep transverse intermetatarsal ligament and tensioned laterally to correct the medial angulation of the second digit (*D*). Postoperative radiograph demonstrating proper alignment of the second digit at the metatarsal-phalangeal joint level following isolated extensor digitorum brevis tendon transfer as well as resection athroplasty of the third, fourth, and fifth digits proximal interphalangeal joints (*E*).

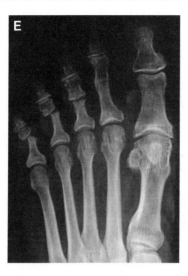

Fig. 7 (*continued*).

interphalangeal joint is prepared for arthrodesis and upon elevating the remaining shaft of the proximal phalanx the plantar plate of the proximal interphalangeal joint is brought into full view. Upon longitudinal sectioning of the plantar plate, the flexor digitorum brevis tendons are easily seen (Fig. 6A). The flexor digitorum longus tendon can then be easily harvested with a hemostat placed between and deep to the medial and lateral slips of the flexor digitorum brevis tendons (Lowell Scott Weil, Sr, DPM, personal communication, 2001) (Fig. 6B). The flexor digitorum longus tendon is then released at this level (Fig. 6C) and split along its central raphe to create medial and lateral tendon slips (Fig. 6D). These tendon slips are transferred deep against the remaining shaft of the proximal phalanx to the dorsal aspect of the base of the proximal phalanx where they are tied into a knot and tensioned to appropriate degree to fully correct the sagittal plane instability (Fig. 6E, G) [52]. If any transverse plane angular deformity is present, the knot can be tensioned in biased fashion (with medial angulation additional tension would be placed laterally to reduce the medial angulation) or the redundant slips can be weaved through the opposite capsule (which has been prepared with a wedge resection to plicate these tissues) to act as a check rein and prevent recurrence of the deformity (with medial angulation the redundant slips would be weaved through the lateral capsule to reduce the medial angulation) (Adam S. Landsman, DPM, PhD, personal communication, 2001). These modifications allow for correction of only mild transverse plane angular deformities [52].

Extensor digitorum brevis tendon transposition is indicated when there is mild to moderate persistent transverse plane angulation [53] following central metatarsal osteotomy. The technique involves transection of the extensor digitorum brevis tendon proximally and rerouting of the tendon from distal to proximal deep

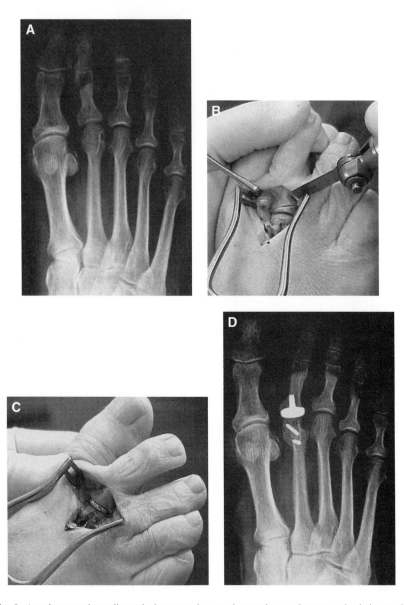

Fig. 8. Anterior-posterior radiograph demonstrating an elongated second metatarsal relative to the adjacent first and third metatarsals as well as medial angulation of the second digit at the metatarsal-phalangeal joint level (*A*). Intraoperative photograph demonstrating laterally biased resection of the base of the proximal phalanx to correct the medial angulation deformity to the second digit (*B*) and following metallic hemi-implant (resurfacing endoprosthesis) insertion (*C*). Significant articular erosion was evident to the second metatarsal head and base of the proximal phalanx at the time of surgery. Postoperative radiograph demonstrating complete correction of the medial angulation deformity of the second digit following medial displacement and shortening Weil metatarsal osteotomy with laterally biased metallic hemi-implant insertion to the base of the proximal phalanx (*D*).

to the deep transverse intermetatarsal ligament where it is either reattached to itself, weaved through the capsule, periosteum, and interosseous musculature, or transferred through a drill hole in the metatarsal shaft and secured to the surrounding soft tissue structures [53] (Fig. 7).

A mini-Akin or Akinette osteotomy of the base of the proximal phalanx is indicated when there is persistent moderate to severe transverse plane angulation [54] following central metatarsal osteotomy. This technique is employed when flexor or extensor tendon transfer has either failed to fully reduce the transverse plane deformity or is not indicated. A transverse osteotomy is performed at the level of the metaphyseal-diaphyseal junction at the base of the proximal phalanx with careful maintenance of the medial (medially angulated digit) or lateral (laterally angulated digit) cortex and periosteum. A second osteotomy is performed distal and oblique to the first to resect a small (1–2 mm) wedge of bone as one would perform an Akin osteotomy to the proximal phalanx of the hallux. The hinge is gently thinned to allow for close approximation of the distal and proximal fragments [54]. If the digit is foreshortened, crescentic-type or opening wedge osteotomies could be employed to maintain the proper digital length pattern. Regardless of the actual osteotomy configuration, if an arthrodesis of the proximal interphalangeal joint has been performed, the fixation can be extended across the osteotomy site to create compression and maintenance of alignment. Simple corrective strapping and compression wrapping of the digit will afford adequate osseous stability and primary healing of the osteotomy without untoward effects.

A metallic hemi-implant endoprosthesis (BIOPRO, Port Huron, Michigan) is indicated in the presence of degenerative joint changes with or without moderate or severe transverse plane pathology. The procedure involves resection of the articular cartilage and a 1-mm section of the underlying subchondral bone plate from the base of the proximal phalanx. If transverse plane malalignment is present, the base of the proximal phalanx is resected in biased fashion to correct the deformity (with medial angulation, more bone is resected laterally and vice versa). A small guide hole is drilled into the center of the base of the proximal phalanx and the implant impacted to lie flush against the remaining subchondral bone (Fig. 8).

Summary

Various central metatarsal osteotomies at the head-neck level have been described in the medical literature, with this article focusing on the minimal incision osteotomy, Weil metatarsal osteotomy and its modifications, and the telescoping metatarsal osteotomy. The indications, surgical techniques, post-operative care, and literature available for each osteotomy have been presented in detail. The use of ancillary lesser digit procedures to aid in sagittal and transverse plane deformity at the lesser metatarsal-phalangeal joint level has also been discussed. The treatment of central metatarsal deformities with head-neck osteotomy with or without concomitant digital procedures is not without complication. Proper preoperative clinical and radiographic analysis; attention to surgical technique; appropriate and aggressive postoperative splinting; and physical therapy should be employed in each instance. Finally, careful patient selection and proper counseling regarding the strong potential to develop well-established complications should be discussed in detail with any prospective patient before performing surgery on the central metatarsals, especially given the significant relief afforded by conservative care measures.

References

[1] Scranton Jr PE. Metatarsalgia: a clinical review of diagnosis and management. Foot Ankle 1981;1(4):229–34.
[2] Trepal MJ, Harkless LB, Jules KT, et al. Central metatarsalgia. Preferred practice guideline. Park Ridge (IL): American College of Foot and Ankle Surgeons; 1998. p. 2–35.
[3] Mann RA, Mann JA. Keratotic disorders of the plantar skin. J Bone Joint Surg [Am] 2003;85(5):938–55.
[4] Mann RA, Mizel MS. Monoarticular synovitis of the metatarsophalangeal joint: a new diagnosis? Foot Ankle 1985;6(1):18–21.
[5] Coughlin MJ. Subluxation and dislocation of the second metatarsophalangeal joint. Orthop Clin N Am 1989;20(4):535–51.
[6] Weinfeld SB. Evaluation and management of crossover second toe deformity. Foot Ankle Clin 1998;3(2):215–28.
[7] Trepal MJ, Harkless LB, Jules KT, et al. Hammer toe syndrome: preferred practice guidelines. J Foot Ankle Surg 1999;38(2):166–78.
[8] Coughlin MJ. Lesser-toe abnormalities. J Bone Joint Surg [Am] 2002;84(8):1446–69.
[9] Holmes GB, Timmerman L. A quantitative assessment of the effect of metatarsal pads of plantar pressures. Foot Ankle 1990;11(3):141–5.
[10] Donahue SW, Sharkey NA. Strains in the metatarsals during the stance phase of gait: implications for stress fractures. J Bone Joint Surg [Am] 1999;81(9):1236–44.
[11] Chang AH, Abu-Faraj ZU, Harris GF, et al. Multistep measurement of plantar pressure alterations using metatarsal pads. Foot Ankle Int 1994;15(12):654–60.
[12] Poon C, Love B. Efficacy of foot orthotics for metatarsalgia. Foot 1997;7(4):202–4.
[13] Postema K, Burn PET, Zande ME, Limbeek JV. Primary metatarsalgia: influence of a custom moulded insole and a rockerbar on plantar pressure. Pros Orthot Int 1998;22(1):35–44.
[14] Viladot A. Metatarsalgia due to biomechanical alterations of the forefoot. Orthop Clin N Am 1973;4(1):165–78.
[15] Smith RW, Reynolds JC, Stewart MJ. Hallux valgus assessment: report of research committee of American orthopaedic foot and ankle society. Foot Ankle 1984;5(2):92–103.
[16] Teitz CC, Harrington RM, Wiley H. Pressures on the foot in pointe shoes. Foot Ankle 1985;5(5):216–21.
[17] Ogilvie-Harris DJ, Carr MM, Fleming PJ. The foot in ballet dancers: the importance of second toe length. Foot Ankle Int 1995;16(3):144–7.
[18] Roukis TS, Jacobs PM, Dawson DD, et al. A prospective comparison of clinical, radiographic, and intra-operative features of hallux rigidus. J Foot Ankle Surg 2002;41(2):76–95.
[19] Bojsen-Møller F. Anatomy of the forefoot, normal and pathologic. Clin Orthop 1980;142:10–8.
[20] Maestro M, Augoyard M, Barouk LS, et al. Biomécaniques et repères radiologiques du sésamoïde latéral de l'hallux par rapport à la palette métatarsienne. Méd Chir Pied 1995; 11(3):145–54.

[21] Barouk LS. Metatarsalgia: metatarsal excess of length in dorso-plantar x-ray view in standing position. In: Forefoot reconstruction. Paris: Springer-Verlag; 2003. p. 214–6.
[22] Maestro M, Besse JL, Ragusa M, Berthonnaud E. Forefoot morphotype study and planning method for forefoot osteotomy. Foot Ankle Clin N Am 2004;8(4):695–710.
[23] Jaworek TE. Intrinsic vascular alterations within osseous tissue of the lesser metatarsals. Arch Podiatr Med Foot Surg 1978;5(2):9–22.
[24] Leemrijse T, Valtin B, Oberlin C. Vascularization of the heads of the three central metatarsals: an anatomical study, its application and considerations with respect to horizontal osteotomies at the neck of the metatarsals. Foot Ankle Surg 1998;4:57–62.
[25] Petersen WJ, Lankes JM, Paulsen F, Hassenpflug J. The arterial supply of the lesser metatarsal heads: a vascular injection study in human cadavers. Foot Ankle Int 2002;23(6):491–5.
[26] Meisenbach RO. Painful anterior arch of the foot: an operation for its relief by means of raising the arch. Am J Orthop Surg 1916;14:206–11.
[27] Schwartz N, Williams Jr JE, Marcinko DE. Double oblique lesser metatarsal osteotomy. J Am Podiatr Assoc 1983;73(4):218–20.
[28] White DL. Minimal incision approach to osteotomies of the lesser metatarsals for treatment of intractable keratosis, metatarsalgia, and tailor's bunion. Clin Podiatr Med Surg 1991;8(1):25–39.
[29] Lauf E, Weinraub GM. Asymmetrical "V" osteotomy: a predictable surgical approach for chronic central metatarsalgia. J Foot Ankle Surg 1996;35(6):550–9.
[30] Kilmartin TE. Distal lesser metatarsal osteotomies: a review of surgical techniques designed to avoid non-union and minimize transfer metatarsalgia. Foot 1998;8(3):186–92.
[31] Idusuyi OB, Kitaoka HB, Patzer GL. Oblique metatarsal osteotomy for intractable plantar keratosis: 10-year follow-up. Foot Ankle Int 1998;19(6):351–5.
[32] Loya K, Guimet M, Rockett MS. Proximal shortening lesser metatarsal osteotomy: a mathematical-geometric basis. J Foot Ankle Surg 2000;39(2):104–13.
[33] Barouk LS. The Weil metatarsal osteotomy. In: Forefoot reconstruction. Paris: Springer-Verlag; 2003. p. 109–32.
[34] Barouk LS. The B.R.T. new proximal metatarsal osteotomy. In: Forefoot reconstruction. Paris: Springer-Verlag; 2003. p. 133–48.
[35] Weil Sr LS. Weil head-neck oblique osteotomy: technique and fixation. Paper presented at Techniques of Osteotomies of the Forefoot. Bordeaux, France, October 20–22, 1994.
[36] Rochwerger A, Launay F, Piclet B, et al. Static instability and dislocation of the second metatarsophalangeal joint: comparative analysis of two different therapeutic modalities. Rev Chir Orthop Rep Appar Mot 1998;84(5):433–9.
[37] Maceira E, Fariñas F, Tena J, et al. Large metatarsal shortenings and post-operative stiffness. Foot Ankle Int 1999;20(10):677–83.
[38] Mühlbauer M, Trnka HJ, Zembsch A, Ritschl P. Short-term outcome of Weil osteotomy in treatment of metatarsalgia. Z Orthop Ihre Grenz 1999;137(5):452–6.
[39] Trnka HJ, Mühlbauer M, Zettl R, et al. Comparison of the results of the Weil and Helal osteotomies for the treatment of metatarsalgia secondary to dislocation of the lesser metatarsophalangeal joints. Foot Ankle Int 1999;20(2):72–9.
[40] Davies MS, Saxby TS. Metatarsal neck osteotomy with rigid internal fixation for the treatment of lesser toe metatarsophalangeal joint pathology. Foot Ankle Int 1999;20(10):630–5.
[41] Vandeputte G, Dereymaeker G, Steenwerckx A, Peeraer L. The Weil osteotomy of the lesser metatarsals: a clinical and pedobarographic follow-up study. Foot Ankle Int 2000;21(5):370–4.
[42] Trnka HJ, Nyska M, Parks BG, Myerson MS. Dorsiflexion contracture after the Weil osteotomy: results of cadaver study and three-dimensional analysis. Foot Ankle Int 2001;22(1):47–50.
[43] Tollafield DR. An audit of lesser metatarsal osteotomy by capital proximal displacement. [Weil osteotomy] Br J Podiatr 2001;4(1):15–9.
[44] Melamed EA, Schon LC, Myerson MS, Parks BG. Two modifications of the Weil osteotomy: analysis on sawbone model. Foot Ankle Int 2002;23(5):400–5.
[45] O'Kane CO, Kilmartin TE. The surgical management of central metatarsalgia. Foot Ankle Int 2002;23(5):415–9.

[46] Leemrijse T, Cadot B, Valtin B, et al. New metacarpal osteotomy: metacarpal cervicocapital shortening osteotomy of the rheumatoid hand. Ann Chir Main Memb Super 1996;15(3):132–7.

[47] Maceira E, Farinas F, Tena J, et al. Analisis de la Rididez Metatarso-falangica en las Osteotomias de Weil. Rev Chir Pied 1998;12(2):35–40.

[48] Johnson JB, Price TW. Crossover second toe deformity: etiology and treatment. J Foot Surg 1989;28(5):417–20.

[49] Pendarvis JA, Mandracchia VJ, Haverstock BD, Granquist JC. A new fixation technique for metatarsal fractures. Clin Podiatr Med Surg 1999;16(4):643–77.

[50] Weil Jr LS. Hammertoe arthrodesis using conical reamers and internal pin fixation. J Foot Ankle Surg 1999;38(5):370–1.

[51] Ford LA, Collins KB, Christensen JC. Stabilization of the subluxed second metatarsophalangeal joint: flexor tendon transfer versus primary repair of the plantar plate. J Foot Ankle Surg 1998;37(3):217–22.

[52] Cohen I, Myerson MS, Weil Sr LS. Flexor to extensor tendon transfer: a new method of tensioning and securing the tendon. Foot Ankle Int 2001;22(1):62–3.

[53] Haddad SL, Sabbagh RC, Resch S, et al. Results of flexor-to-extensor and extensor brevis tendon transfer for correction of the crossover second toe deformity. Foot Ankle Int 1999;20(12):781–8.

[54] Davis WH, Anderson RB, Thompson FM, Hamilton WG. Proximal phalanx basilar osteotomy for resistant angulation of the lesser toes. Foot Ankle Int 1997;18(2):103–4.

ELSEVIER
SAUNDERS

Clin Podiatr Med Surg
22 (2005) 223–245

CLINICS IN
PODIATRIC
MEDICINE AND
SURGERY

The Tailor's Bunionette Deformity: A Field Guide to Surgical Correction

Thomas S. Roukis, DPM

Weil Foot and Ankle Institute, 1455 East Golf Road, Suite 131, Des Plaines, IL 60016, USA

The term "tailor's bunionette" is derived from the position of a sitting tailor with legs crossed, which places abnormal pressure on the lateral aspect of the fifth metatarsal head [1]. This term is used to describe a constellation of symptoms or deformities involving the fifth metatarsal and fifth metatarsal-phalangeal joint and is characterized by a symptomatic prominence of the fifth metatarsal head with or without rotational deformities to the fifth digit [2]. The actual symptoms are varied and can involve the dorsal, lateral, and plantar aspects of the fifth metatarsal head [2].

Although the actual incidence and prevalence of tailor's bunionette deformity in the general population is not known, several retrospective studies indicate that the condition is between 3 and 10 times more common in women than men and has a peak incidence during the fourth and fifth decades of life [3–6]. Although treatments such as oral anti-inflammatories, corticosteroid injections, topical linements, and physical therapy may resolve any associated bursitis or fifth metatarsal-phalangeal joint synovitis, and the use of periodic débridement and topical keratolytics may limit the degree of keratotic buildup, these measures will not likely provide any long-term relief in the presence of a structural fifth metatarsal deformity [1,2]. Similarly, conservative measures such as shoe-gear changes, orthoses, and various forms of pressure-dispersion padding (orthodigita) may lessen the symptomatology associated with a painful structural tailor's

E-mail address: troukis@footankledeformity.com

0891-8422/05/$ – see front matter © 2005 Elsevier Inc. All rights reserved.
doi:10.1016/j.cpm.2004.10.004

podiatric.theclinics.com

bunionette deformity but they have not been shown to provide any long-term measurable relief and are best considered palliative in nature [2].

Etiology

The etiology of the tailor's bunionette deformity is varied but involves a series of anatomical or structural abnormalities to the fifth metatarsal head or shaft. These variations can be specifically defined as a (1) true tailor's bunionette (dorsal, lateral, or combined prominence to the fifth metatarsal head with associated buritis or keratotic lesions secondary to shoe-gear irritation about a "dumbbell shaped" fifth metatarsal head); (2) plantar-displaced fifth metatarsal (excessive sagittal plane declination of the fifth metatarsal with associated bursitis or keratotic lesions secondary to chronic and repetitive pressure during gait); (3) lateral or plantar fifth metatarsal head condyle exostosis (true osseous enlargement as a result of traction enthesiopathy or chronic pressure induced irritation); (4) a splayfoot deformity (transverse plane widening of the forefoot with an increased intermetatarsal 1–2 and 4–5 angle or lateral bowing of the fifth metatarsal shaft); and (5) a combination of one or more of the above deformities (see references [2,5,8–12]). Additional influences include (1) biomechanical dysfunction (fifth ray instability or fixed forefoot or rearfoot varus deformities); (2) congenital structural deformities; (3) connective tissue disease or inflammatory arthridities; (4) fifth metatarsal-phalangeal joint trauma (ruptured collateral ligaments); (5) neuromuscular disorders resulting in a rigid cavus or cavo-varus forefoot posture; and (6) iatrogenic causes [2].

Clinical examination

The clinical examination should include a through assessment of the patient's past and present medical history, with special emphasis placed on the chronicity of the symptoms, effect of the condition on their activities of daily living and employment responsibilities, and progression of the deformity [2]. A detailed evaluation of the foot, ankle, and lower leg concentrating on the presence of any keratotic lesions, adventitial bursa formation, fifth metatarsal-cuboid joint and fifth metatarsal-phalangeal joint range of motion, global forefoot posture, and palpation of the periarticular structures to determine areas of maximum symptomatology and exostosis formation should be performed [1,2]. The use of specialized pressure gait analysis and imaging examinations (MRI, CT scan, bone scan, fluoroscopy, musculoskeletal ultrasound, and arthrography) are useful when faced with a particularly difficult or multilevel deformity but should not be used with regularity given the expense of these tests and paucity medical literature to support their routine use [2]. Weight-bearing radiographs, however, are essential, and when combined with the clinical examination will allow complete evaluation in all but the most severe or unusual abnormities involving the fifth metatarsal and fifth metatarsal-phalangeal joint [8,9,12].

Radiographic analysis

Weight-bearing anterior-posterior and lateral radiographs in the angle and base of gait should be made of both feet if pathology exists bilateral or of the symptomatic foot with any necessary comparison views of the contralateral uninvolved foot to allow for full evaluation of the structural alignment and osseous morphology about the forefoot and specifically the fifth metatarsal (see references [2,8,9,12]).

The significant radiographic measurements that define a tailor's bunionette deformity include the (1) intermetatarsal 4–5 angle (angle formed between the longitudinal bisection of the fourth metatarsal and the medial cortex of the fifth metatarsal; normal, less than 8°) [8,9,12]; (2) fifth metatarsal-phalangeal angle (degree of medial deviation of the fifth digit in relation to the longitudinal bisection of the fifth metatarsal; normal, less than 10°) [9,11,12]; (3) lateral deviation angle or lateral bowing (angle formed between the medial cortex of the fifth metatarsal and bisection of the fifth metatarsal head and neck; normal, less than 3°) [8,12]; (4) fifth metatarsal lateral prominence distance (protrusion of the lateral metatarsal head surface from the shaft measured from a line drawn along the lateral cortex of the fifth metatarsal shaft and another line drawn along the lateral cortex of the fifth metatarsal head; normal, less than 4 mm) [9,12]; (5) 4–5 metatarsal head distance (distance between the lateral cortex of the fourth metatarsal head and the medial cortex of the fifth metatarsal head; normal, less than 3 mm) [13]; and (6) fifth metatarsal plantar-declination angle (horizontal bisection of the fifth metatarsal in relation to the weight-bearing surface; normal, 10°) [2]. The normal length of the fifth metatarsal is considered to be 12 mm shorter than the fourth metatarsal to allow for a gentle oblique taper from the central metatarsals in a lateral direction [14]. Finally, the normal width of the fifth metatarsal head is considered less than 13 mm [12]. When combined with the patient's medical history, physical demands, and clinical examination, appropriate determination of these angular and linear measurements can help aide in selection of the appropriate surgical procedure [2].

Metatarsal head ostectomy

Resection of the lateral one quarter to one third of the fifth metatarsal head has been advocated for the surgical treatment of the tailor's bunionette deformity [2,15,16]. This procedure has been termed an "ostectomy," "exostectomy," "condylectomy," or "simple bunionectomy" and can be performed in isolation or as part of other surgical techniques. Fifth metatarsal head ostectomy as an isolated procedure is indicated when hypertrophy of the dorsal or lateral aspect of the fifth metatarsal head region without soft tissue or structural deformity of the fifth metatarsal is deemed the primary pathology or when the patient is considered an inappropriate candidate for more complex procedures (Fig. 1A) [2,15,16].

The surgical technique begins with the patient positioned in the supine position on the operating room table with a well-padded bolster placed beneath the ipsilateral buttock to control the physiologic external rotation of the lower limb. Following local anesthesia alone or combined with intravenous sedation, the foot and ankle is exsanguinated with an elastic bandage and an ankle tourniquet inflated for hemostasis. A lateral or, less commonly, a dorsal incision measuring 2 to 3 cm in length is then placed directly overlying the fifth metatarsal head from the base of the proximal phalanx to the metatarsal neck. The author prefers a lateral incision placed at the junction between the dorsal and plantar skin rather than a dorsal incision for several reasons. First, the incision respects the vascular supply to the fifth metatarsal region and allows for easy mobilization of the abductor digiti minimi, which can be covered with a simple split-thickness skin graft should wound healing complications arise [17,18]. Second, the incision lies in a "safe zone" so that dissection directly to bone with the elevation of full-thickness skin flaps can be performed which limits unnecessary dissection and associated prolonged postoperative edema and scar tissue formation [18]. Third, all of the pertinent anatomy lies at the lateral aspect of the fifth metatarsal head region and is easily accessible with a direct lateral incision approach, which also affords significant exposure of the dorsal and plantar aspects of the fifth metatarsal head should these areas need to be exposed. Finally, as the skin incision matures it will contract and, rather than pulling the fifth digit dorsally as would happen with a dorsal approach, the fifth digit will be held in corrected position or slightly abducted, which limits the development of a hammer toe contracture. With these issues in mind, the incision is deepened directly through the skin, superficial fascia, and adipose to the level of the capsule and periosteum overlying the fifth metatarsal head and fifth metatarsal-phalangeal joint. The capsule and periosteum is then reflected using a surgical scalpel and periosteal elevator to expose the lateral aspect of the fifth metatarsal head and neck as well as a limited amount of the dorsal and plantar aspects of the fifth metatarsal head. The insertion of the abductor digiti minimi onto the plantar-lateral aspect of the base of the proximal phalanx is either left intact (no adduction deviation of the fifth digit present) or dissected free for later advancement and repair (adduction deviation present). The lateral one quarter to one third of the fifth metatarsal head is then resected in line with the lateral border of the foot, rather than in line with the fifth metatarsal shaft, using power instrumentation (Fig. 1B). The author prefers to use power instrumentation to take advantage of the thermal necrosis that occurs with this technique to limit late postoperative osseous regrowth. Alternatively, a hand-held osteotome and mallet may be used to sculpt the lateral aspect of the fifth metatarsal head and the raw bone surface cauterized with an electrocautery unit to achieve the same outcome. The lateral aspect of the fifth metatarsal head is resected in line with the lateral border of the foot rather than the lateral aspect of the fifth metatarsal shaft to create a smooth lateral surface

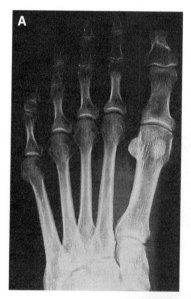

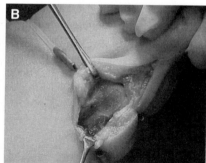

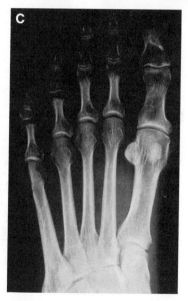

Fig. 1. Anterior-posterior radiograph of a symptomatic tailor's bunionette with concomitant fourth and fifth hammer toe formation. Note the enlarged dumbbell-shaped fifth metatarsal head without significant increase in the intermetatarsal 4–5 or lateral deviation angles (*A*). Intraoperative photograph following lateral ostectomy of the fifth metatarsal head. Note that the fifth metatarsal head and shaft have been resected in line with the lateral border of the foot rather than the lateral aspect of the fifth metatarsal shaft (*B*). Anterior-posterior radiograph following lateral ostectomy to the fifth metatarsal head with resection arthroplasty of the fourth and fifth digit proximal interphalangeal joints (*C*).

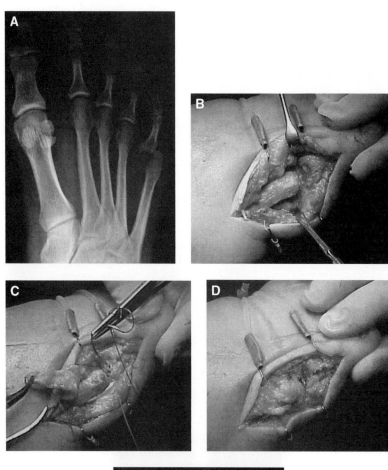

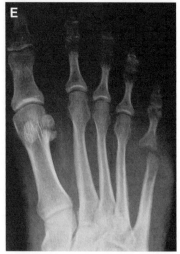

overlying the fifth metatarsophalangeal joint region (Fig. 1C) [16]. Following irrigation of the surgical site, the fifth digit is held in a slightly overcorrected abducted and plantarflexed position and the abductor digiti minimi tendon is reattached either directly to the surrounding deep tissues or through a small drill hole in the base of the proximal phalanx. The remaining deep tissues and skin edges are reapproximated using the surgeon's preferred technique, although a running subcuticular suture and adhesive bandage application will allow earlier bathing and negate the need to remove sutures at a later date.

This simple technique allows for immediate weight bearing in a bulky, well-padded surgical dressing and postoperative shoe. Because the author uses absorbable sutures and adhesive bandages to support the incision edges, the initial surgical dressings are routinely removed at 7 to 10 days and the patient placed in a roomy athletic or oxford shoe without weight-bearing restrictions. The patient is allowed to bathe and shower after the initial dressings are removed and instructed to leave the adhesive dressings alone until they come off with wear. The patient is allowed to return to activities as soon as the pain subsides and is seen on regular intervals to assess the incision site healing and any other related issues.

The use of this technique as an isolated procedure was initially advocated by Davies in 1949 [15]. Since then, few modifications of the actual surgical procedure have been presented [2,10,16]. These modifications include resection of the base of the proximal phalanx of the fifth toe, the plantar condyle to the fifth metatarsal head, and any associated adventitial bursa formation [2,10,16]. Unfortunately, no detailed outcome analysis of the fifth metatarsal head ostecomy procedure has been published in the literature. The author has found this to be a valuable procedure when combined with a resectional arthroplasty of the fifth digit proximal interphalangeal joint to treat a combined fifth digit hammer toe and mild to moderate tailor's bunionette deformity due to a widened fifth metatarsal head with or without exostosis formation.

Metatarsal head resection

Resection of the fifth metatarsal head with or without soft tissue interposition is indicated when an ostectomy or osteotomy are contraindicated [2,19,20].

Fig. 2. Anterior-posterior radiograph following a failed lateral ostectomy of the fifth metatarsal head. Note that the lateral aspect of the fifth metatarsal head has been incorrectly resected in line with the lateral aspect of the fifth metatarsal shaft and the fifth digit is dislocated from the fifth metatarsal-phalangeal joint (A). Intraoperative photograph following resection of the fifth metatarsal head and deepening of the phalangeal base concavity (B). The abductor digiti minimi has been released and reflected proximally (held in hemostat on left), and multiple sutures have been passed through several drill holes in the remaining fifth metatarsal neck-shaft segment (suture held in needle driver to right) (C). The abductor digiti minimi has been interposed between the remaining fifth metatarsal neck shaft and base of the proximal phalanx (D). Anterior-posterior radiograph following resection arthroplasty with abductor digit minimi interposition. Note the increased joint space and realigned fifth metatarsal-phalangeal joint relationship (E).

Situations where this may be appropriate include severe osteopenia, extensive degenerative joint changes, chronic ulceration with or without osteomyelitis, previous failed surgery, or poor medical health (Fig. 2A) [2,19,20].

The surgical technique begins as described previously with the patient positioned in the supine position on the operating room table with a well-padded bolster placed beneath the ipsilateral buttock. Following local anesthesia alone or combined with intravenous sedation, the foot and ankle is exsanguinated with an elastic bandage and an ankle tourniquet inflated for hemostasis. A lateral or, less commonly, a dorsal incision measuring 2 to 3 cm in length is then placed directly overlying the fifth metatarsal head from the base of the proximal phalanx to the metatarsal neck. The incision is deepened directly through the skin, superficial fascia, and adipose to the level of the capsule and periosteum overlying the fifth metatarsal head and metatarsophalangeal joint. The capsule and periosteum is then reflected using a surgical scalpel and periosteal elevator to expose the entire fifth metatarsal head and neck circumferentially. Using a power saw, the fifth metatarsal head is transected at the surgical neck level in a biased fashion to resect slightly more bone laterally and plantarly to avoid pressure-related issues from osseous prominence in these areas (Fig. 2B). The author prefers to "spear" the metatarsal head with a small-diameter threaded Kirschner wire, which is used as a toggle to manipulate the osseous fragment and facilitate any additional dissection necessary to extirpate the bone without undue soft tissue injury. Following irrigation of the surgical site, the abductor digiti minimi tendon is transected from the base of the proximal phalanx with sharp dissection and interposed within the resected joint space (Fig. 2C). The tendon is stabilized with several small 1.5-mm drill holes through the remaining metatarsal for a secure and snug fit, and the remaining portion on the base of the proximal phalanx is then sutured to the lateral aspect of the interposed tendon to properly balance the fifth metatarsophalangeal joint (Fig. 2D).

This technique has several advantages over leaving the void unfilled or "hourglassing" the capsule and periosteum as has been commonly described [2,19,20]. First, the abductor digiti minimi tendon is thick and robust and can readily fill the dead space created by excision of the metatarsal head and will limit the amount of fifth toe contracture, resulting in an improved cosmetic result. Second, the interposition of tendon around the remaining fifth metatarsal will limit the amount of bleeding from the raw end of bone and, therefore, the potential to develop a hematoma. Third, interposing the tendon and securely suturing the tendon through several small drill holes creates a stable, well-balanced joint complex that does not require the use of axial Kirschner wire placement (Fig. 2E). This allows early unrestricted weight bearing in a standard postoperative shoe, bathing, and return to shoe gear after the first postoperative visit. It also obviates the need to remove the wire at a later date. Finally, because the long extensor and flexor tendons are left untouched, their function is undisturbed, which is not the case with the hourglassing technique that encircles whatever tissue is available, including the regional tendons, and limits their proper function [2,19,20]. The remaining deep tissues and skin edges are then reapproximated using the surgeon's preferred technique, although a running subcuticular suture and adhesive bandage application will allow earlier bathing and negate the need to remove sutures at a later date.

This simple technique allows for immediate weight bearing in a bulky, well-padded surgical dressing and postoperative shoe. The patient is allowed to bathe and shower after the initial dressings are removed and instructed to leave the adhesive dressings alone until they come off with wear. The patient is allowed to return to activities as soon as the pain subsides and is seen on regular intervals to assess the incision site healing and any other related issues.

Dorris and Mandel [20] performed a retrospective review of 50 such procedures in 34 patients for severe, recurring keratotic lesions to the plantar aspect of the fifth metatarsal head. Despite a 59% incidence of fifth digit malalignment (dorsal contracture or proximal retraction), only 3% developed a symptomatic transfer lesion [20]. The use of a silicone prosthetic implant has been described in the literature as being useful in the presence of a high degree of fifth digit instability following resection of the fifth metatarsal head [2,21]. Addante et al [21], in a retrospective review of 50 fifth metatarsal-phalangeal joint silicone prosthetic implant arthroplasty, found a complication rate of 16%, including the development of symptomatic transfer lesions and recurrence of the deformity. When combined with the known problems of metatarsal-phalangeal joint silicone implant arthroplasty, this technique is not considered appropriate for routine use [2].

Minimal incision (percutaneous) osteotomy

Minimal incision or percutaneous osteotomy of the fifth metatarsal has received little attention in the literature [22]; however, the author finds this a valuable procedure for treating fifth metatarsal plantar or, less commonly, lateral diabetic neuropathic ulcerations recalcitrant to, or recurrent despite, appropriate conservative measures.

The surgical technique begins with the patient positioned in the supine position on the operating room table with a well-padded bolster placed beneath the ipsilateral buttock. The use of an ankle tourniquet is optional and not routinely employed because of the limited soft tissue dissection afforded by this procedure. Following local anesthesia alone or combined with intravenous sedation, a 1-cm vertical incision is placed through the skin at the lateral aspect of the fifth metatarsal surgical neck and dissected down to the level of the capsule and periosteum using a hemostat with the jaws fully closed. Once the bone is directly palpated, the hemostat jaws are opened with one jaw placed dorsally and one plantarly until the hemostat can be advanced from lateral to medial. This elevates the soft tissue from the lateral, dorsal, and plantar aspects of the fifth metatarsal surgical neck. Under direct image intensification, a power saw is used to create an osteotomy from lateral to medial and biased from distal to proximal with a slight dorsal shelf existing between the capitol fragment and remaining metatarsal to limit dorsal displacement. However, if a plantar lesion is present, the osteotomy should be performed directly from medial to lateral to allow for some dorsal migration of the plantar capitol fragment. Following completion of the osteo-tomy, a small osteotome is inserted to verify completion of the osteotomy and to pry the capitol fragment medially to correct the relative 4–5 intermetatarsal angle or dorsally to elevate the fifth metatarsal head in the sagittal plane. The resultant lateral osseous prominence remaining on the proximal fifth metatarsal is then resected with a small Rongeur or, less commonly, a small hand-held or power rasp. Percutaneous Kirschner wire or breakaway-type pins can be used to stabilize the osteotomy but are usually not necessary. The surgical site is irrigated, and the skin is closed with a single absorbable suture. A light dressing is applied, and the patient is placed directly back into an athletic-type shoe or roomy oxford with full weight bearing to tolerance allowed. The initial surgical dressings are removed in 7 to 10 days, and the patient placed back into their regular shoe gear as tolerated.

White [22], in a limited retrospective review of 40 fifth metatarsal minimal incision unfixated osteotomies as described above, found no delayed unions, one (3%) malunion, and two (5%) nonunions. Although performed through an open incision technique, Catanzariti et al [23] performed a retrospective review of 38 similar nonfixated fifth metatarsal osteotomies and found no nonunions but a 26% incidence of lesion recurrence and 35% incidence of transfer lesions. These authors concluded that the routine use of this osteotomy should be avoided because of the significant incidence of sagittal plane malunion [23]. Zvijac et al [24], in a similar retrospective review of 50 open-incision nonfixated fifth meta-tarsal osteotomies, found no nonunions, a mean dorsal displacement of 3 mm, and mean of 2 mm of shortening. Unfortunately, there was no mention of the incidence of lesion recurrence or transfer metatarsalgia [24].

Pontius et al [25] performed a retrospective review comparing fixated (N = 22) and nonfixated (N = 34) distal fifth metatarsal osteotomies of varying con-figurations with the majority being similar to the procedure described in this section. The nonfixated group had a statistically significant increased incidence of dorsal displacement (mean 2 mm) and shortening (mean 2.7 mm). They concluded that the use of internal fixation provides a more predictable healing pattern, degree of correction, and less dorsal displacement and shortening [25]. Based on the literature, this technique is probably a poor choice for routine use in those patients presenting with a tailor's bunionette or prominent plantar condyle and no medical comorbidities. However, the significant dorsal displacement and shortening achieved with this procedure as well as the limited soft tissue dissection necessary are ideal in the diabetic-compromised host. This procedure, when combined with early and aggressive shoe-gear alteration (rocker sole modifications) and multidensity custom orthoses, will rapidly and predictably resolve a recalcitrant or recurrent neuropathic ulceration about the fifth metatarsal head with minimal complications and avoid the need for more aggressive, costly, and complicated soft tissue and osseous reconstruction techniques.

Metatarsal head-neck osteotomies

Distal fifth metatarsal head-neck osteotomies are considered efficacious for correction of mild to moderate transverse and sagittal plane deformities (see references [2,5–7,13,14,26–29]). Though a myriad of techniques have been described (peg-in-hole, chevron, crescentic, inverted-L, oblique), this section focuses on two osteotomies: the reverse Scarf and distal oblique osteotomy (see references [13,14,28,29]).

The surgical technique for either osteotomy begins with the patient positioned in the supine position on the operating room table with a well-padded bolster placed beneath the ipsilateral buttock. Following local anesthesia alone or combined with intravenous sedation, the foot and ankle is exsanguinated with an elastic bandage and an ankle tourniquet inflated for hemostasis. A lateral or, less commonly, a dorsal incision measuring 2 to 3 cm in length is then placed directly overlying the fifth metatarsal head from the base of the proximal phalanx to the metatarsal neck. The incision is deepened directly through the skin, superficial fascia, and adipose to the level of the capsule and periosteum overlying the fifth metatarsal head and metatarsophalangeal joint. The capsule and periosteum is then reflected using a surgical scalpel and periosteal elevator to expose the dorsal, lateral, and plantar aspects of the fifth metatarsal head and neck.

In a reverse-Scarf osteotomy, a power saw is used to make an oblique osteotomy in the horizontal plane, outlined from dorsal-distal to plantar proximal over the exposed fifth metatarsal head-neck and distal shaft region with slight plantar angulation if one wishes to plantar transpose the metatarsal capitol fragment or, conversely, with slight dorsal angulation if one wishes to elevate the distal capitol fragment (Fig. 3A) [14,28]. A 90° dorsal-distal osteotomy is performed just proximal to the fifth metatarsal head articular cartilage, and then a 45° proximal-plantar osteotomy is performed at the proximal extent of the original horizontal osteotomy (Fig. 3B). A small osteotome is placed between the plantar capitol fragment and the metatarsal shaft and gently rotated to verify completion of the osteotomy. The fifth metatarsal shaft is grasped with a small clamp (ie, phalangeal clamp) and pried laterally, while at the same time the plantar capitol fragment is displaced medially with a small osteotome or forcep until the desired amount of correction is achieved (Fig. 3C). This is the so-called "push-pull" maneuver. The plantar capitol fragment is then provisionally stabilized with a small clamp or smooth Kirschner-wire and intraoperative image intensification is used to verify complete correction of the deformity and determine the appropriate level of fixation. Two small-diameter non-lag screws or threaded Kirschner wires are placed to maintain the reduction. Non-lag screws are used because the configuration of the osteotomy is inherently stable but prone to troughing with large medial displacement of the plantar capitol fragment, and the screws are simply used to maintain reduction rather than compress the osteotomy fragments (Fig. 3D). The redundant lateral head, neck, and shaft is resected with power instrumentation and smoothed to a normal anatomical contour with a hand-held rasp or power rotary burr (Fig. 3E). If troughing occurs, or if one wishes to further plantar-displace the capitol fragment, the redundant lateral bone shelf can be resected before final fixation and inserted in between the horizontal portion of the osteotomy. Conversely, if one wishes to further dorsally angulated the capitol fragment, a small distally based wedge of bone can be resected from the plantar capitol fragment, as this is the deeper of the two fragments, and the capitol fragment elevated to the desired level.

A distal oblique osteotomy is performed much like the Weil metatarsal osteotomy for the central metatarsals but with intentional maintenance of the proximal plantar cortical-periosteal hinge [13,29,30] (Fig. 4A). The osteotomy

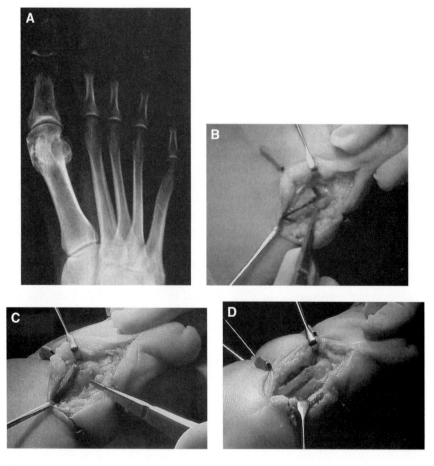

Fig. 3. Anterior-posterior radiograph of a splay-foot deformity (increased intermetarsal 1–2 and 4–5 angles) with an increased fifth metatarsal lateral deviation angle (*A*). Intraoperative photograph following reverse-Scarf fifth metatarsal osteotomy (*B*) revealing the degree of medial translation obtained (*C*). Final appearance following resection of the redundant dorsal and lateral hyperostosis (*D*). Anterior-posterior radiograph following Lapidus-Akin bunionectomy and reverse-Scarf fifth metatarsal osteotomy fixated with "no-profile" internal fixation. Note the degree of medial translation and correction of lateral bowing achieved (*E*).

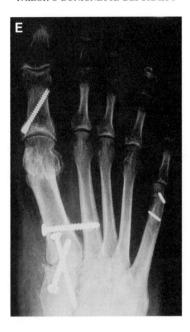

Fig. 3 (*continued*).

begins at a level 2 mm below the dorsal articular cartilage of the fifth metatarsal head and is angled proximally is such a manner as to extend to the junction of the distal and middle one third of the fifth metatarsal (Fig. 4B, C). The plantar-proximal cortical-periosteal junction is gently "feathered" in such a fashion as to allow motion between the dorsal and plantar capitol fragments but not result in two completely separate fragments. The "push-pull" maneuver is performed as described previously, with the exception that the plantar capitol fragment is displaced medially through rotation about the proximal-plantar cortical-periosteal hinge rather than direct medially displacement as the fragments are still connected proximally (Fig. 4D). The plantar capitol fragment is provisionally stabilized and intraoperative image intensification is used to verify complete correction of the deformity and determine the appropriate level of fixation. Two small-diameter nonlag screws or threaded Kirschner wires are placed to maintain the reduction for the reasons described previously. The redundant lateral head, neck, and shaft is resected in line with the lateral border of the foot with power instrumentation (Fig. 4E) and smoothed to a normal anatomical contour with a hand-held rasp or power rotary burr (Fig. 4F, G). Following irrigation of the surgical site, the fifth digit is held in a slightly overcorrected abducted and plantarflexed position and the abductor digiti minimi tendon is reattached either directly to the surrounding deep tissues or through a small drill hole in the base of the proximal phalanx if it had been released during the initial dissection. The remaining deep tissues and skin edges are reapproximated using the surgeons preferred technique, although a running subcuticular suture and adhesive bandage

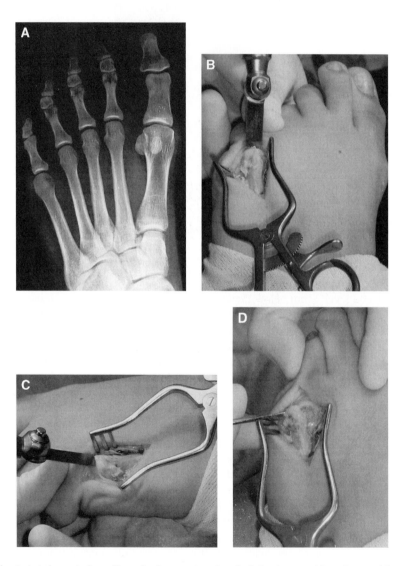

Fig. 4. Anterior-posterior radiograph of a symptomatic tailor's bunionette with an increased lateral deviation angle (*A*). Intraoperative photographs demonstrating the proper location and orientation of the distal oblique osteotomy in the anterior-posterior (*B*) and lateral (*C*) planes. Intraoperative photograph following completion of the osetotomy and the "push-pull" maneuver demonstrating the degree of correction obtained (*D*). Following rigid internal fixation, the redundant dorsal and lateral hyperostosis before (*E*) and after (*F*) resection and remodeling. Anterior-posterior radiograph following distal oblique fifth metatarsal osteotomy revealing complete reduction of lateral bowing (*G*).

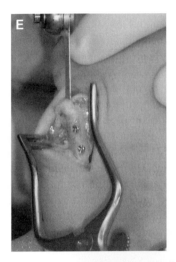
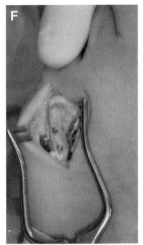

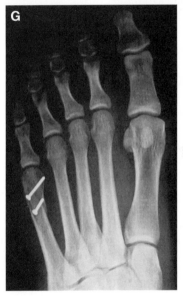

Fig. 4 (*continued*).

application will allow earlier bathing and negate the need to remove sutures at a later date.

Both of these techniques allow for immediate weight bearing in a bulky, well-padded surgical dressing and postoperative shoe. The patient is allowed to bathe and shower after the initial dressings are removed and instructed to leave the adhesive dressings alone until they come off with wear. The patient is allowed to return to activities as soon as the pain subsides and is seen at regular intervals to assess the incision site healing and any other related issues.

Seide and Petersen [28], in a retrospective review of 10 reverse Scarf osteotomies with a minimum of 1-year follow-up, determined a mean intermetatarsal 4–5 angle reduction of 3.5° (10.3–6.8°). These authors concluded that the reverse Scarf osteotomy allows for significant reduction of the intermetatarsal 4–5 angle and, due to its inherent stability, allows for immediate weight bearing without fear of sagittal plane malunion. Unfortunately, no other published articles regarding the outcomes of this technique are available beyond a simple technique guide described by Barouk [14].

Schabler et al [13] performed a retrospective review of 24 distal oblique osteotomies with a minimum 3-year follow-up, determined a mean intermetatarsal 4–5 reduction of 4.5° (10.5–6.0°); a mean lateral deviation angle reduction of 8.4° (10.2–1.8°); and a mean 4–5 metatarsal head distance reduction of 3.2 mm (4.9–1.7 mm). The authors concluded that the configuration of the osteotomy affords inherent stability and prevention of undesired sagittal plane malalignment and excessive shortening due to the intact plantar proximal cortical-periosteal hinge [13].

Metatarsal shaft osteotomies

Fifth metatarsal shaft osteotomies are considered effective for correction of moderate transverse and sagittal plane deformities [2,31]. The main type of fifth metatarsal shaft osteotomy described is the long oblique wedge resection or "mini-Juvara" osteotomy [31].

The surgical technique begins with the patient positioned in the supine position on the operating room table with a well-padded bolster placed beneath the ipsilateral buttock. Following local anesthesia alone or combined with intravenous sedation, the foot and ankle is exsanguinated with an elastic bandage and an ankle tourniquet inflated for hemostasis. A dorsal incision measuring 4 to 5 cm in length is then placed directly overlying the fifth metatarsal neck and shaft from the fifth metatarsal to the junction between the proximal and middle one third of the fifth metatarsal. The incision is deepened directly through the skin, superficial fascia, and adipose to the level of the capsule and periosteum overlying the fifth metatarsal neck and shaft. The capsule and periosteum is then reflected using a surgical scalpel and periosteal elevator to expose the dorsal and medial aspects of the fifth metatarsal neck and shaft. Using a power saw, a long oblique osteotomy with the sagittal plane is outlined from distal-medial to proximal-lateral and performed in such a manner as to maintain the proximal-lateral cortical-periosteal hinge. A small 2- to 3-mm medially based wedge of bone is then resected from the proximal and medial portion of the fifth metatarsal and the proximal-lateral hinge gently "feathered" as described previously. A small bone clamp is used to close the osteotomy, which medially rotates the distal fifth metatarsal capitol fragment. If any gapping is present between the distal and proximal capitol fragments, the prominence between the two fragments can be resected with reciprocal planning (used if additional correction in necessary to fully reduce the deformity) or the small wedge of bone resected could be morselized and packed within the gap as an autogenous bone graft (used if no additional correction is necessary). An image intensifier is used to verify complete reduction of the deformity before performing final fixation with a small, oblique screw oriented from distal-lateral to proximal-medial at the junction between 90° to the osteotomy and 90° to the fifth metatarsal shaft. Following irrigation, the author prefers to advance the interosseous musculature in a dorsal and lateral direction to cover the osteotomy with well-perfused vascular muscle to enhance the healing potential of this type of osteotomy. The fifth digit is held in a slightly over-corrected abducted and plantarflexed position, and the deep tissues and skin edges are reapproximated using the surgeon's preferred technique, although a running subcuticular suture and adhesive bandage application will allow earlier bathing and negate the need to remove sutures at a later date.

This technique does not allow for immediate weight bearing because of the orientation and fragility of the osteotomy and, therefore, should be protected in either a formal short-leg non–weight-bearing cast or removable immobilization boot. Because the skin is closed with absorbable sutures and adhesive bandages, the author prefers to use a removable immobilization boot, which allows the initial surgical dressings to be removed at 7 to 10 days—at which point the patient is allowed to bathe and shower. Serial radiographs are obtained to monitor osseous healing and, once verified through clinical (no edema and no pain on stress range of motion to the osteotomy site) and radiographic parameters (primary osseous healing without callus formation), the patient is allowed to return to a roomy athletic or oxford shoe with weight bearing to tolerance. The patient should be seen on regular intervals to assess the incision site healing and any other related issues.

Castle et al [31], in a retrospective review of 26 long oblique wedge resection osteotomies, found a mean intermetatarsal 4–5 angle reduction of 1.5° (7.9–6.4°) and a mean lateral deviation angle reduction of 3.9° (4.1–0.2°). One osteotomy fractured following a traumatic incident in the early postoperative period but there were no reported incidences of delayed union, malunion, or transfer lesions [31]. This osteotomy appears most useful for the correction of an abnormal lateral deviation angle rather than increased intermetatarsal 4–5 angle.

Metatarsal base osteotomies

Proximal fifth metatarsal base osteotomies are used to reduce significantly increased intermetatarsal 4–5 angles or when a great degree of sagittal plane correction is desired because of the longer lever-arm afforded by the proximal location of the osteotomy (see references [2–4,32–36]). The osteotomy configurations described include closing and opening base wedges, crescentic, and chevron shaped in the sagittal and transverse planes (see references [2–4,32–34]). However, the tenuous vascular supply in the proximal base region about the metaphyseal-diaphyseal junction where these osteotomies are by definition performed, and the inherent instability, reserves them for use in only the most clearly defined instances [2,35].

The surgical technique begins with the patient positioned in the supine position on the operating room table with a well-padded bolster placed beneath the ipsilateral buttock. Following local anesthesia alone or combined with intravenous sedation, the foot and ankle is exsanguinated with an elastic bandage and an ankle tourniquet inflated for hemostasis. A dorsal incision measuring 3 to 4 cm in length is then placed directly overlying the fifth metatarsal base within the proximal one third of the fifth metatarsal. The incision is deepened directly through the skin, superficial fascia, and adipose to the level of the capsule and periosteum overlying the fifth metatarsal base. The capsule and periosteum is

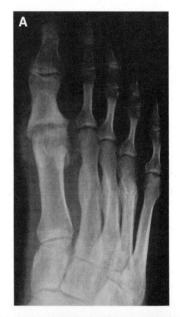

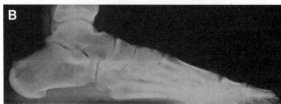

Fig. 5. Anterior-posterior (A) and lateral (B) radiographs following a first metatarsal-phalangeal joint modified-Cheilectomy, resultant sequential second, third, and fourth metatarsal stress fractures, and persistent pain and deformity about the first metatarsal-phalangeal joint and plantar aspect of the fifth metatarsal head. Anterior-posterior (C) and lateral (D) radiographs following first metatarsal-phalangeal joint capsule-periosteum interpositional implant arthroplasty and B.R.T. dorsiflexory fifth metatarsal osteotomy.

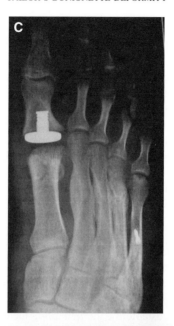

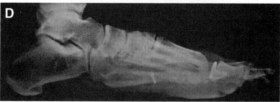

Fig. 5 (*continued*).

then reflected using a surgical scalpel and periosteal elevator to expose the dorsal and medial aspects of the fifth metatarsal shaft and base. Using a power saw, a short oblique osteotomy within the sagittal plane is outlined from distal-medial to proximal-lateral and performed in such a manner as to maintain the proximal-lateral cortical-periosteal hinge. A small 1- to 2-mm medially based wedge of bone is then resected from the proximal and medial portion of the fifth metatarsal, and the proximal-lateral hinge gently "feathered" as described previously. A small bone clamp is used to close the osteotomy, which medially rotates the distal fifth metatarsal capitol fragment. If any gapping is present between the distal and proximal capitol fragments, the prominence between the two fragments can be resected through reciprocal planning or the small wedge of bone resected could be morselized and packed within the gap as an autogenous bone graft for the reasons previously described. Alternatively, a crescentic osteotomy within the sagittal plane or a chevron osteotomy within the transverse plane could be performed. The distal capitol fragment created by either osteotomy is then rotated medially and, if desired, within the sagittal plane to fully correct the deformities present. Regardless of the osteotomy employed, an image intensifier is used to verify complete reduction of the deformity before performing final fixation with a small, oblique screw oriented from distal-lateral to proximal-medial or multiple smooth Kirchner wires connecting the fifth and fourth metatarsals and oriented within the horizontal plane are placed and left either prominent beneath the skin or exposed for later removal.

If the deformity is strictly within the sagittal plane, a B.R.T. (Barouk-Rippstein-Toulec) osteotomy can be performed [14]. This is a long oblique dorsiflexory wedge osteotomy that involves removal of a thin (1 mm) dorsal-distally based wedge of bone with gentle "feathering" of the cortical-periosteal hinge (Fig. 5A, B). The osteotomy is fixated with a low-profile lag screw (Fig. 5C, D). Following irrigation, the author prefers to advance the interosseous musculature in a dorsal and lateral direction to cover the osteotomy with well-perfused vascular muscle to enhance the healing potential of this type of osteo-tomy. The remaining deep tissues and skin edges are reapproximated using the surgeon's preferred technique, although a running subcuticular suture and adhesive bandage application will allow earlier bathing and negate the need to remove sutures at a later date.

Except for the B.R.T. osteotomy, the remaining techniques does not allow for immediate weight bearing because of the orientation and fragility of the osteo-tomy and, therefore, should be protected in a formal short-leg non–weight-bearing cast if percutaneous Kirchner wire fixation was performed or a removable immobilization boot if buried fixation was employed. The author prefers to use buried fixation if possible with a removable immobilization boot, which allows the initial surgical dressings to be removed at 7 to 10 days, at which point the patient is allowed to bathe and shower. Serial radiographs are obtained to monitor osseous healing, and once verified, the patient is allowed to return to a roomy athletic or oxford shoe with weight bearing to tolerance after the per-cutaneous Kirschner wires have been removed. The patient is seen at regular intervals to assess the incision site healing and any other related issues as pre-viously described.

Gerbert et al [32] described a preliminary report on the use of a closing base wedge osteotomy to the fifth metatarsal in 20 feet with "very favorable results." Following this initial description, a similar procedure termed the "D.R.A.T.O." or "derotational, angulational transposition osteotomy" was retrospectively reviewed by Buchbinder [3] in 38 feet with a minimum follow-up of 3 years. Delayed union occurred in 13%, transfer lesions developed in 13%, malunion occurred in 8%, and recurrence of the original lesion developed in 5% [3]. Diebold and Bejjani [4], in a retrospective review of 12 proximal fifth metatarsal base chevron osteotomies fixated with several horizontally oriented transfixtion Kirschner wires between the fifth and fourth metatarsals, determined a mean intermetatarsal 4–5 angle reduction of 10° (18–8°) with no incidence of non-union, malunion, or transfer lesions. Diebold [34], in a retrospective review of 22 proximal fifth metatarsal base chevron osteotomies fixated with several hori-zontally oriented transfixtion Kirschner wires between the fifth and fourth meta-

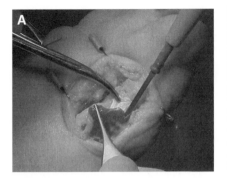
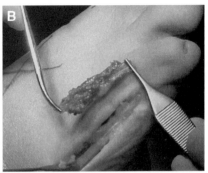

Fig. 6. Intraoperative photograph during (A) and following (B) abductor digiti minimi "myoectomy." Note the use of electrocautery for dissection (A) and the reduction of the "pseudo-tailor's bunionette" achieved (B).

tarsals with a minimum follow-up of 3 years, determined a mean intermetatarsal 4–5 angle reduction of 10.8° (12.1–1.3°) with no incidence of nonunion, malunion, or transfer lesions. The authors concluded that the significant stability afforded by "transmetatarsal pinning" over crossed fixation of the osteotomy alone was responsible for the lack of malunions and nonunions experienced in their studies [4,34,36]. Nothing beyond the surgical technique has been published regarding the B.R.T. osteotomy [14].

Ancillary soft tissue procedures

In certain select instances the abductor digit minimi is hypertrophied and creates the illusion of a "pseudo-tailor's bunionette" about the lateral border of the fifth metatarsal [37]. In these rare instances, a "myoectomy" of the lateral portion of the abductor digiti minimi (superficial to the tendon) may be performed to remove the muscular prominence. This is used in conjunction with, and following completion of, the osseous and capsule-tendon balanced procedures described previously. An electrical cautery probe is used to dissect the abductor digit minimi from the underlying tendon that allows for appropriate hemostatsis to reduce the incidence of hematoma formation (Fig. 6A). The end result is a more cosmetically appealing lateral border of the foot without compromised fifth metatarsal-phalangeal joint function as most of the abductor digiti minimi muscle remains intact from origin to insertion (Fig. 6B).

Summary

Surgical intervention of the tailor's bunionette deformity is simple to perform, provides significant reduction of preoperative patient symptoms, and appears to be resistant to significant complications, regardless of the surgical procedure performed. Early guarded weight bearing, the use of low-profile, small-diameter internal fixation, and protection of the surrounding soft tissue supportive structures should be employed to ensure a successful outcome with minimal complications if the level and fixation techniques employed allow.

References

[1] Mann RA, Coughlin MJ. Keratotic disorders of the plantar skin. In: Mann RA, Coughlin MJ, editors. Surgery of the foot and ankle. 6th edition. St. Louis: Mosby; 1993. p. 441–65.

[2] American College of Foot and Ankle Surgeons. Tailor's bunion and associated fifth metatarsal conditions: preferred practice guidelines. Park Ridge (IL): American College of Foot and Ankle Surgeons; 1993.

[3] Buchbinder IJ. DRATO procedure for tailor's bunion. J Foot Surg 1982;21(3):177–9.

[4] Diebold PF, Bejjani FJ. Basal osteotomy of the fifth metatarsal with intermetatarsal pinning: a new approach to the tailor's bunion. Foot Ankle 1987;8(1):40–5.

[5] Steinke MS, Boll KL. Hohmann-Thomasen metatarsal osteotomy for tailor's bunion (bunionette). J Bone Joint Surg [Am] 1989;71(3):423–6.

[6] Hansson G. Sliding osteotomy for tailor's bunion: brief report. J Bone Joint Surg [Br] 1989; 71(2):324.

[7] Heckman JD, Harkless LB, Wirth MA, Higgins KR. The Sponsel oblique fifth metatarsal osteotomy: evaluation with long-term follow-up. Foot 1991;1(1):37–44.

[8] Fallat LM, Bucholz J. Analysis of the tailor's bunion by radiographic and anatomic display. J Am Podiatr Assoc 1980;70(12):597–603.

[9] Nestor BJ, Kitaoka HB, Ilstrup DM, et al. Radiologic anatomy of the painful bunionette. Foot Ankle 1990;11(1):6–11.

[10] Fallat LM. Pathology of the fifth ray, including the tailor's bunion deformity. Clin Podiatr Med Surg 1990;7(4):689–715.

[11] Coughlin MJ. Etiology and treatment of the bunionette deformity. Instr Course Lect 1990;39:37–48.

[12] Karasick D. Preoperative assessment of symptomatic bunionette deformity: radiologic findings. Am J Radiol 1995;164(1):147–9.

[13] Schabler JA, Toney M, Hanft JR, Kashuk KB. Oblique metaphyseal osteotomy for the correction of tailor's bunions: a 3-year review. J Foot Surg 1992;31(1):79–84.

[14] Barouk LS. Some pathologies of the fifth ray: tailor's bunion. In: Barouk LS, editor. Forefoot reconstruction. Paris: Springer-Verlag; 2002. p. 276–83.

[15] Davies H. Metatarsus quintus valgus. BMJ 1949;1:664–5.

[16] Kitaoka HB, Holiday AD. Lateral condylar resection for bunionette. Clin Orthop 1992;278: 183–92.

[17] Attinger C, Cooper P, Blume P, Bulan E. The safest surgical incisions and amputations applying the angiosome principles and using Doppler to assess the arterial-arterial connections of the foot and ankle. Foot Ankle Clin N Am 2001;6(4):745–99.

[18] Papp CT, Hasenöhrl C. Small toe muscles for defect coverage. Plast Reconstr Surg 1990;86(5): 941–5.

[19] Lelièvre J. Exostosis of the head of the fifth metatarsal bone. Concours Med 1956;78:4815–6.

[20] Dorris MF, Mandel LM. Fifth metatarsal head resection for correction of tailor's bunions and sub-fifth metatarsal head keratoma: a retrospective analysis. J Foot Surg 1991;30(3):269–75.

[21] Addante JB, Chin M, Makower BL, et al. Surgical correction of tailor's bunion with resection of fifth metatarsal head and Silastic sphere implant: an 8-year follow-up study. J Foot Surg 1986; 25(4):315–20.

[22] White DL. Minimal incision approach to osteotomies of the lesser metatarsals: For treatment of intractable keratosis, metatarsalgia, and tailor's bunion. Clin Podiatr Med Surg 1991;8(1):25–39.

[23] Catanzariti AR, Friedman C, DiStazio J. Oblique osteotomy of the fifth metatarsal: a five year review. J Foot Surg 1988;27(4):316–20.

[24] Zvijac JE, Janecki CJ, Freeling RM. Distal oblique osteotomy for tailor's bunion. Foot Ankle 1991;12(3):171–5.

[25] Pontious J, Brook JW, Hillstrom HJ. Tailor's bunion: Is fixation necessary? J Am Podiatr Med Assoc 1996;86(2):63–73.

[26] Frankel JP, Turf RM, King BA. Tailor's bunion: clinical evaluation and correction by distal metatarsal osteotomy with cortical screw fixation. J Foot Surg 1989;28(3):237–43.

[27] Friend G, Grace K, Stone HA. L-osteotomy with absorbable fixation for correction of tailor's bunion. J Foot Ankle Surg 1993;32(1):14–9.

[28] Seide HW, Petersen W. Tailor's bunion: results of a scarf osteotomy for the correction of an increased intermetatarsal IV/V angle: a report of ten cases with a 1-year follow-up. Arch Orthop Trauma Surg 2001;121(3):166–9.

[29] Sakoff M, Levy AI, Hanft JR. Metaphyseal osteotomy for the treatment of tailor's bunions. J Foot Surg 1989;28(6):537–41.

[30] Barouk LS. The Weil lesser metatarsal osteotomy. In: Barouk LS, editor. Forefoot reconstruction. Paris: Springer-Verlag; 2002. p. 109–32.

[31] Castle JE, Cohen AH, Docks G. Fifth metatarsal distal oblique wedge osteotomy utilizing cortical screw fixation. J Foot Surg 1992;31(5):478–85.

[32] Gerbert J, Sgarlato TE, Subotnick SI. Preliminary study of a closing wedge osteotomy of the fifth metatarsal for correction of a tailor's bunion deformity. J Am Podiatr Assoc 1972;62(6):212–8.

[33] Shrum DG, Sprandel DC, Marshall H. Triplanar closing base wedge osteotomy for tailor's bunion. J Am Podiatr Med Assoc 1989;79(3):124–7.

[34] Diebold PF. Basal osteotomy of the fifth metatarsal for the bunionette. Foot Ankle 1991;12(2):74–9.

[35] Shereff MJ, Yang QM, Kummer FJ, et al. Vascular anatomy of the fifth metatarsal. Foot Ankle 1991;11(6):350–3.

[36] Massengill JB, Alexander H, Parson JR, Schecter MJ. Mechanical analysis of Kirschner wire fixation in a phalangeal model. J Hand Surg 1979;4(4):351–6.

[37] Carmont MR, Bruce C, Bass A, Carty H. An accessory abductor muscle of the fifth toe? An unusual cause of a lump in the foot. Foot Ankle Surg 2002;8:125–8.

ELSEVIER
SAUNDERS

Clin Podiatr Med Surg
22 (2005) 247–264

CLINICS IN
PODIATRIC
MEDICINE AND
SURGERY

Midfoot Osteotomies for the Cavus Foot

Thomas W. Groner, DPM,
Lawrence A. DiDomenico, DPM, FACFAS*

*Department of Podiatric Surgery, Forum Health/Northside Medical Center, 500 Gypsy Lane,
Youngstown, OH 44501, USA*

Midfoot osteotomies have long been used for a wide variety of congenital and acquired deformities. These deformities include such entities as metatarsus adductus, clubfoot, arthritis, and pes cavus. Severe pes cavus often necessitates some form of midfoot osteotomy. In 1940, Cole popularized a dorsiflexory wedge osteotomy through the lesser tarsus to correct a cavus-type condition [1]. Japas later proposed a midfoot V-shaped osteotomy [2]. Through the years, several modifications and new techniques have been published. This article serves as an overview of documented and lesser-known techniques for the treatment of pes cavus with midfoot osteotomies. The etiology, evaluation, classification, and various treatments for pes cavus are also discussed.

Pes cavus

Pes cavus can be defined as an abnormal elevation of the medial longitudinal arch. Historically, the condition was synonymous with being born into nobility. Ancient Chinese culture used binding techniques to create shortened, high-arched feet [3]. In 1853, Little first coined the term "pes cavus" [4]. Presently, pes cavus is often secondary to a neuromuscular disorder and associated muscle imbalance. The condition may be classified as neuromuscular, congenital, idiopathic, or traumatic. A study by Brewerton reviewed 77 patients with pes cavus [5]. Three quarters of the patients were found to have an underlying neuromuscular condition, and congenital and idiopathic etiologies were reported at 14% and 11%

* Corresponding author.
E-mail address: ld5353@aol.com (L.A. DiDomenico).

respectively. The most common condition was Charcot-Marie-Tooth, followed by meningomyelocele and poliomyelitis [5]. Numerous other etiologies may underly the cavus foot. These include diseases of the spinal cord such as tumors, syringomyelia, spinal muscular atrophy, and poliomyelitis [4,6,7]. Other neuro-muscular conditions are muscular dystrophy, cerebral palsy, Friedreich's ataxia, Roussy-Levy syndrome, Dejerine-Sottas syndrome, and spina bifida [4,5,7–11]. Traumatic cases may include severe burns, malunion of fractures, compartment syndrome, and crush injuries [7,12–14]. Congenital disorders, such as syphilis, lymphedema, arthrogryphosis, and clubfoot, have also been reported [4,6,7, 13,15]. The cavus foot rarely presents before the age of 3 but may progress depending on the etiology [16]. It is important to perform a thorough neurologi-cal evaluation at the first sign of pathology to prevent a delay in diagnosis.

Evaluation and classification

A complete history is the basis of any patient encounter, but it is of the utmost importance when a patient has pes cavus. It is important to obtain a birth history and family history and to inquire about any developmental delays [17]. In the pediatric population a cavus foot should be considered a sign of a neuromuscu-lar disorder until proven otherwise. Treatment of any underlying disease should take precedence over treatment of the foot deformity [18].

In adults, examination of the cavus foot may or may not yield any neurologic or muscular abnormalities. The presenting complaint is often pain or weakness in the arch, fatigue, ankle joint instability, heel pain, or pain under the metatarsal heads. As the deformity worsens, the amount of the foot that comes in contact with the ground decreases and the remaining weight-bearing areas are subjected to increased pressure. As a result, the patient often shows signs of callus plan-tar to the metatarsal heads [7]. Plantar callus can lead to ulceration in the neu-ropathic individual.

When ankle joint instability is the presenting complaint the amount of heel varus should be recognized (Fig. 1). Heel varus will increase as the cavus foot progresses, therefore leading to recurrent ankle sprains and instability. One must remember that with rearfoot varus the midtarsal joint is locked and subtalar joint pronation is limited [6]. A thorough gait examination may go a long way in aiding with the diagnosis. Furthermore, excessive wear on the lateral aspect of shoes may be noted. After gait analysis, a manual muscle examination should be performed.

Manual muscle testing aids in the identification of imbalance between strong and weak muscles. In neuromuscular disease, weakness of a muscle group results in overpowering by that muscle's antagonist. Agonist and antagonist muscles should be tested. Anterior muscles will oppose the triceps surae. The anterior tibialis muscle is the antagonist of the peroneous longus, whereas the posterior tibialis opposes the peroneous brevis muscle. In a study by Tynan [19], it was

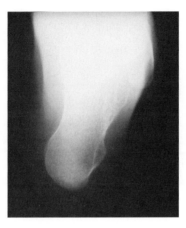

Fig. 1. Calcaneal axial radiographic view of rigid hindfoot varus.

noted that patients with a cavus deformity usually have a dominant peroneous longus compared with a weak anterior tibialis. Often, in Charcot-Marie-Tooth for example, the peroneous brevis and anterior tibialis muscles are weak. This leads to unopposed pull by the posterior tibialis and peroneous longus respectively. Hansen has coined the latter process "peroneal longus overpull" [12]. Progression of these imbalances leads to calcaneal varus, forefoot adduction, and plantarflexion of the first ray. The degree of muscle imbalance will become paramount if surgery is later performed [7,20].

Another aspect of the clinical examination for a patient with pes cavus is the block test. Coleman and Chestnut [21] popularized the test as a simple way to evaluate the flexibility of the hindfoot. The test is performed by placing the lateral border of the foot on an elevated block. The medial aspect of the foot is suspended off the block and as the patient attempts to bear weight the rearfoot is assessed. Surgical treatment of the rearfoot is unnecessary if it is flexible. If it is a rigid deformity, then surgical treatment may include the forefoot and rear-foot [17,21,22].

The next step in the evaluation of pes cavus is radiographic assessment. A weight-bearing lateral view is especially helpful (Fig. 2). Several radiographic angles may be obtained to help evaluate the apex of maximum deformity. The calcaneal inclination angle measures the plantar aspect of the calcaneous with the weight-bearing surface. Normal measurement is around 25 degrees, and anything over 30 degrees should be considered a moderate deformity. The long axes of the talus and first metatarsal create Meary's angle. A normal measurement is 0 to 5 degrees, but one study found an average of 18 degrees in patients with Charcot-Marie-Tooth [17,23,24]. Hibb's angle is formed by the axis of the first metatarsal with the body of the calcaneous. Barenfield [25] suggested a lesser-known calcaneometatarsal angle formed by the long axis of the first metatarsal with the axis of the calcaneous. Normal value is said to be less than 140 degrees with a decreased measurement in the cavus foot [25,26].

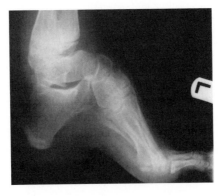

Fig. 2. Weight-bearing lateral radiographic view with severe increase in calcaneal inclination angle.

Pes cavus may be classified not only as flexible and rigid but also according to the findings of the radiographic evaluation. In anterior cavus the apex of the deformity is at either Lisfranc's or Chopart's joint. Meary's angle would be greater than 10 degrees and the calcaneal inclination would be less than 30 degrees. Posterior cavus has an apex of deformity proximal to Chopart's joint. Meary's angle is less than 10 degrees while calcaneal inclination is greater than 30 degrees. It is not unusual for both anterior and posterior deformities to be present. If this is the case, the patient is classified as having a combined cavus foot type. Further classification exists depending on the extent of the anterior cavus. For example, if the first metatarsal is plantarflexed alone in relation to the midtarsal and subtalar joints, this is classified as anterior local cavus. On the other hand, if all metatarsals are plantarflexed it is an anterior global deformity [27].

Finally, a complete evaluation may include a few other ancillary tests. Electromyography accompanied with nerve conduction velocity studies may be requisite based on the patient's neurological examination. In rare cases, muscle and nerve biopsy may be required for identification of various neurologic disorders [7]. Biopsies are usually performed only when clinical, radiographic, and electrodiagnostic studies fail to discern the underlying entity [6].

Associated conditions

Several associated conditions may be present in the cavus foot. Contracted digits are one of the most common accompanying deformities. The typical contracture of the toes seen in the cavus foot led early authors on the subject to describe the deformity as clawfoot [1]. Hammertoe-type deformities in pes cavus are often caused by extensor substitution. In extensor substitution the extensor digitorum longus muscle overpowers the lumbricales during swing phase and causes dorsiflexion and retrograde buckling at the metatarsal phalangeal joints. In the cavus foot this may be precipitated by loss or weakness of the anterior tibialis muscle.

Because the weight-bearing surface of the foot is in essence decreased in the cavus foot, patients are prone to developing metatarsalgia and plantar heel pain. Heel pain may be due to plantar fascitis or contracture, but often it is simply the result of contusion conditions from the increased force of weight bearing [12].

There are several other conditions or components of pes cavus that must be mentioned. For example, the plantarflexed first ray is an excessively plantarflexed first metatarsal relative to metatarsals 2 through 5. Forefoot valgus is described as an everted forefoot relative to the rearfoot when the subtalar joint is in neutral. Conversely, forefoot varus is described as an inverted forefoot relative to the rearfoot in subtalar joint neutral position. Next, rearfoot varus is an inverted position of the calcaneous compared with the weight-bearing surface while in subtalar joint neutral position [4]. Also, metatarsus adductus may be present concomitantly with pes cavus (Fig. 3) [28]. At our institution, a transverse plane midfoot osteotomy is used to correct any accompanying adductus when performing cavus reconstruction.

Surprisingly, equinus may be an associated condition of pes cavus. It is manifested as an overpowering of the posterior muscles, often with accompanied weakness of the anterior muscles, which leads to decreased ankle joint dorsiflexion. It may occur in patients with neuromuscular disorders, such as Charcot-Marie-Tooth, muscular dystrophy, and spina bifida. It is common to see spastic equinus with cerebral palsy. Pseudoequinus is not a true equinus but it is a

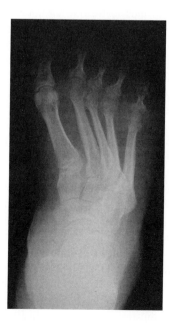

Fig. 3. Severe metatarsus adductus as an associated condition of cavus deformity.

condition that occurs when the ankle joint functions as if there is an equinus deformity. Pseudoequinus is common in rigid anterior pes cavus. The patient's foot dorsiflexes in an attempt to get the heel to the floor. This compensation may lead to an increased calcaneal inclination angle. The remaining inability of the ankle to dorsiflex during weight bearing is termed "pseudoequinus." Long-standing pseudoequinus in the cavus foot may sometimes result in spurring at the talar navicular joint. When a bony blockage leads to limitation of ankle dorsiflexion, osseous equinus occurs [4,29].

Conservative treatment

According to Mosca [18], there is little role for nonoperative treatment of the cavus foot because deformities are progressive in nature and severe by the time of presentation. An attempt should be made initially at conservative treatment. Patients with mild deformities will benefit most from conservative treatment. Operative treatment may be appropriate if there is an underlying medical condition. Nonsurgical treatment may be as simple as palliative care in the form of hyperkeratosis debridement. Further conservative care should consist of physical therapy, accommodative shoes, and orthoses.

Physical therapy may consist of daily stretching exercises for the Achilles tendon and plantar fascia. These stretches are not unlike those routinely pre-scribed for patients with plantar fascitis. Stretching helps maintain suppleness in the arch of the foot and aids in treating an equinus deformity. Dwyer [16] advocated plantar fascia stretching in conjunction with a metatarsal bar for cavus deformities [17]. Aggressive physical therapy is especially important in neuro-muscular diseases such as cerebral palsy. Treatment in cerebral palsy should begin at an early age and combine daily stretching with splinting and bracing. Muscle strengthening exercises will aid in gait stability of the cavus foot.

Accommodative shoes are another aspect of conservative treatment. Custom-made shoes are especially important in neuropathic patients to prevent ul-cerations. Shoes can be accommodated to unload undue pressure at the heel and metatarsal heads. Materials such as PPT and Plastizote provide cushioning and limit shear forces [7].

It is important to provide the patient with some form of an orthotic device. Inserts and ankle-foot-orthoses may be used in conjunction with custom-made shoes. Patients with a rigid plantarflexed first ray and a flexible hindfoot may benefit from an orthotic with a medial forefoot post that helps eliminate hindfoot inversion [23]. A solid or articulated ankle-foot-orthotic can provide needed stability in a patient with significant deformity. It is extremely important that individuals are carefully fitted with these devices to prevent breakdown of the skin while providing the proper stability. When dispensing any type of orthotic, remember that periodic adjustments will most likely be necessary due to the progressive nature of most deformities.

Surgical intervention

Indications for surgical correction include pain, progressive deformity, and ankle instability. The goals of surgery are to balance muscle forces, correct deformities, and provide a mobile plantigrade foot [17,18]. It is important not only to determine the apex of the deformity but to address the entire deformity. No single procedure or algorithm can be used exclusively to correct pes cavus. Surgical correction consists of soft tissue and osseous procedures. Soft tissue releases and tendon transfers are useful for flexible deformities and as adjuncts to osseous procedures. In the actively growing pediatric patient, osseous procedures may not be acceptable, but remember that soft tissue procedures will not correct rigid deformities. The progressive nature of many neurologic conditions will make soft tissue correction temporary at best [27]. Because of the myriad of etiologies and associated deformities, a wide variety of surgical techniques are necessary to correct the symptomatic cavus foot.

Soft tissue procedures

Initial soft tissue procedures include plantar fascial release and Steindler stripping. Thomas [30] first reported using plantar fasciotomies for pes cavus. Later, the procedure was used alone for correction of cavus deformity caused by clubfoot and polio [31]. Today it is used primarily as an adjunct to osseous procedures. Steindler stripping is a release of the plantar fascia coupled with release of the plantar intrinsic musculature [32,33]. Typically, the abductor hallucis, abductor digiti quinti, and flexor digitorum brevis are stripped from the calcaneous. Modifications have been reported to avoid injury to the plantar neurovascular structures [7,34]. Regardless of the exact procedure, the calcaneal inclination angle should theoretically decrease with release of the windlass mechanism.

Tendon transfers

Tendon transfers are used to correct flexible deformities. A muscle should not be transferred unless its strength is at least grade 4 of 5, as transferred tendons will lose one grade in strength [35]. Transfers include the peroneous longus, posterior tibialis, and anterior tibialis. Peroneous longus transfer is indicated for a flexible plantarflexed first ray, and it is useful for any condition that causes a weak anterior tibialis muscle and dropfoot. Transfer of the peroneous longus not only eliminates first metatarsal plantarflexion but aids in dorsiflexion of the ankle [36]. Similarly, other augmentations of the peroneous longus may be useful in correcting a flexible plantarflexed first ray. These include lengthening as well as transfer or tenodesis to the peroneous brevis to combat excess plantarflexion.

Posterior tibialis tendon transfer can be risky because it is an out-of-phase transfer. Despite this, with proper physical therapy the procedure is useful for the treatment of dropfoot and a weak anterior tibialis muscle. The procedure reduces the deformity and also allows the patient to function better without bracing. If the individual acquires an equinus component then a gastrocnemius recession or Achille's lengthening may be necessary at the time of transfer [36].

In the inverted foot, if the anterior tibialis muscle remains strong, the tendon can be split and transferred laterally. This will aid in ankle dorsiflexion and decrease swing phase supination. Careful evaluation of anterior tibialis muscle strength should be performed before undertaking this procedure.

Another well-known soft tissue procedure is the Jones tenosuspension. The extensor hallucis longus tendon is transferred proximally from the hallux to the first metatarsal to correct plantarflexion. The procedure also consists of arthrodesis of the hallux interphalangeal joint. The extensor hallucis longus functions as an ankle dorsiflexor while metatarsal phalangeal joint extension is eliminated [37]. Similar surgical techniques, such as a modified Hibb's procedure, consist of transfer of the extensor digitorum longus to the lateral cuneiform, cuboid, or lesser metatarsals [38]. These transfers are indicated for flexible anterior cavus and correction of concomitant hammertoe deformities.

Osseous procedures

Soft tissue procedures are used for flexible deformities, and osseous correction is warranted for correction of rigid cavus foot deformities. Most osseous surgical procedures are used in conjunction with other procedures. A first metatarsal dorsiflexory wedge osteotomy is useful for treatment of a rigid plantarflexed first ray. Callus under the plantar aspect of the first metatarsal is a symptom of this fixed deformity. At our institution, a single 3.5-mm cortical screw is preferred for internal fixation. Another technique is to fixate the wedge with a three- or four-hole one-quarter or one-third tubular plate along with 2.7-mm or 3.5-mm cortical screws [39].

A Lapidus procedure may also be performed to allow for the appropriate amount of dorsiflexory correction. This surgical approach may be especially useful in the presence of metatarsus varus and marked neuromuscular disease [4,12]. McElvenny and Caldwell [40] initially recommended first metatarsal cuneiform joint arthrodesis to remedy anterior cavus by elevating and supinating the metatarsal. First metatarsal cuneiform arthrodesis may be fixated with 3.5-mm cortical or 4.0-mm cortical or cancellous screws with or without a plate. Again, cancellous bone may be used as a shear-strain relief bone graft across the joint to combat micromotion [41]. In some instances, anterior cavus may be corrected with multiple metatarsal osteotomies. A three-incisional approach should be employed over the base of the first metatarsal and between the bases of the second and third as well as the fourth and fifth metatarsals respectively.

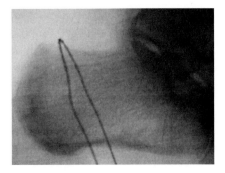

Fig. 4. Placement of percutaneous giggly saw just before through-and-through calcaneal osteotomy.

Jahss [42] described a truncated wedge arthrodesis of the tarsometatarsal joint for fixed anterior cavus. The procedure is essentially a Lis Franc's joint arthrodesis. The base of the wedge is wider at the dorsal aspect compared with plantar, and the forefoot is elevated out of its plantarflexed attitude. The procedure should not be used to correct subtalar or rearfoot pathology. As with any cavus reconstruction, determining the apex of the deformity is mandatory. Overzealous resection of the wedge or excision distal to the apex of the deformity can lead to a postoperative rocker-bottom foot [4].

A calcaneal osteotomy is indicated in the presence of rigid hindfoot varus. The Coleman block test should be performed to be certain that the varus position of the calcaneous is not reducible. We prefer a percutaneous displacement osteotomy of the calcaneous and believe that fixation is best accomplished with a pair of parallel percutaneous 7.3-mm cannulated screws driven from posterior-inferior to anterior-superior across the osteotomy site. An alternative to the percutaneous osteotomy is the Dwyer lateral closing wedge osteotomy. These can be performed with the standard open technique or in a percutaneous fashion (Fig. 4); the former method can be used with the aid of a giggly saw (Fig. 5) [43]. Dwyer believed that a plantar fascial release was a supplemental requirement

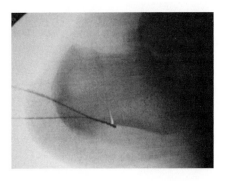

Fig. 5. Giggly saw technique immediately after performing calcaneal osteotomy. Two 7.3-mm cannulated screws were then driven from posterior to anterior across the osteotomy site.

[44]. Similarly, the authors perform a plantar fasciotomy or Steindler stripping as an adjunctive procedure. A preponderance of ankle equinus as a result of ankle plantarflexors overpowering the anterior muscles is common. A tendo-Achilles lengthening or gastrocnemius recession is performed under these circumstances.

Triple arthrodesis is a common procedure for correction of severe pes cavus with associated arthrosis. It is also useful as a salvage procedure in skeletally mature adolescents with rigid pes cavus [17,35,45]. With proper wedge resection, triple arthrodesis is a powerful technique that can correct all three planes of deformity.

Midfoot osteotomies

Midfoot osteotomies are useful in reducing rigid anterior cavus deformities. Several variations have been used over the years to enhance correction. Regardless of the level, plane, or technique of the midfoot osteotomy, the aforementioned adjunctive procedures aid in the complete correction of the deformity.

Cole procedure

Cole [1] described a closing wedge osteotomy with removal of a dorsally based wedge. The wedge is removed from a distal cut through the cuboid and cuneiforms coupled with a proximal cut through the cuboid and navicular. This elevates the forefoot out of equinus. Although Cole is credited with popularizing the procedure, it was first described by Saunders 5 years earlier [15]. The Cole procedure is indicated for rigid anterior pes cavus when the apex of the deformity

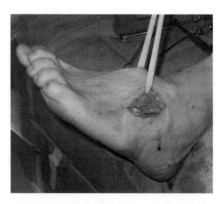

Fig. 6. Cole procedure soft tissue dissection of lateral incision.

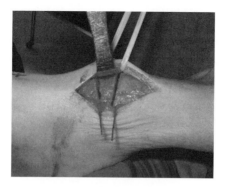

Fig. 7. An approximately 1-cm dorsally based wedge. The medial aspect of the wedge can be made wider to address associated metatarsus adductus.

is located at the midfoot. It is contraindicated when the apex of the deformity is any place other than the midfoot [1,46]. Also, the procedure is not indicated for the skeletally immature foot, as this can lead to shortening. It is important that the talonavicular and calcaneal-cuboid joints are spared during this procedure. In addition, an osteotomy with a wider medial wedge has been proposed as a modification for multiplanar correction or more often a wider lateral wedge is used to address adduction [47].

The Cole midfoot osteotomy has been employed with one-, two-, and three-incision approaches [46]. We prefer a two-incision approach (Fig. 6). A medial incision is extended from the first metatarsal cuneiform joint to the navicular. A lateral incision is placed over the cuboid. Care is taken to use blunt dissection to avoid the dorsalis pedis artery and the anterior tibialis tendon with the medial incision and the sural nerve with the lateral. A power saggital saw or a long oscillating saw is then used for the osteotomy. The dorsal base should be approximately 1 cm wide (Fig. 7). The apex of the wedge should meet at the plantar aspect of the navicular and cuboid (Fig. 8). At this time, associated

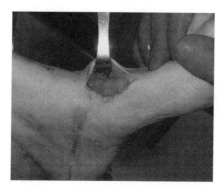

Fig. 8. Reduction of midfoot osteotomy after wedge removal.

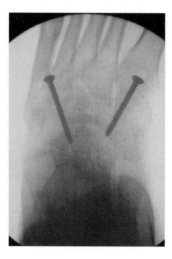

Fig. 9. AP radiograph after reduction and fixation of midfoot osteotomy.

metatarsus adductus can be combated by making the lateral aspect of the wedge wider. A Steindler stripping is necessary to aid in dorsiflexion of the osteotomy site. Fixation may consist of any combination of Steinman pins, staples, and screws. Care must be taken when using screws that the surrounding joint spaces are not violated. Some surgeons prefer to use screws in combination with a quarter tubular plate [39]. We prefer 3.5-mm cortical screws for fixation (Figs. 9 and 10). Fixation is stable with postoperative weight bearing because of the benefit of ground reactive forces across the osteotomy site. Weight bearing to tolerance with a cast and crutches is usually allowable after only a few weeks. At about 4 weeks the cast may be replaced by a Cam Walker until bone healing is complete.

A recent study by Wulker and Hurchler [48] reported satisfaction in eight of 11 patients who required a dorsal closing wedge osteotomy for pes cavus. Of the

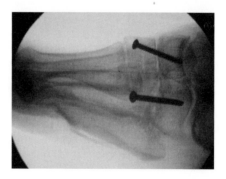

Fig. 10. Cole midfoot osteotomy lateral radiographic view after screw fixation.

patients not satisfied with the outcome of surgery, two went on to a nonunion and the third required subsequent Achille's tendon lengthening to correct an underlying equinus deformity [48]. Furthermore, a gastrocnemius recession or Achille's lengthening is often necessary to correct the equinus deformity before osseous reconstruction of the midfoot.

Japas midfoot osteotomy

Japas [2] described a through-and-through V-shaped osteotomy that was designed to circumvent shortcomings of the Cole procedure, such as shortening of the foot. The technique is indicated for anterior pes cavus and serves to elevate the forefoot into a more rectus position. It is not advised in the immature foot. The tranverse plane V-shaped osteotomy is performed with the apex proximal in the navicular and the arms extending distally through the cuboid and the first cuneiform respectively [2]. A single dorsal longitudinal incision is most often used. Steinman pins are the most common form of fixation.

An advantage of this procedure is that a wedge need not be removed, and therefore the foot does not shorten. However, the disadvantages outweigh this advantage. The Japas procedure can often lead to arthrosis and delayed union [4]. Also, the patient may be left with an uncomfortable hump that is created on the dorsal aspect of the foot. It is our belief that the Cole procedure is easier, more reliable, and has fewer complications.

Midtarsal dome osteotomy

Wilcox and Weiner [26] advocated an alternative approach for correction of rigid anterior cavus. The results of the subsequent study demonstrated a 94% satisfaction rate in patients older than 8 years of age, but only 42% satisfactory results were obtained in patients younger than 8 [26]. The procedure is indicated when the apex of the deformity lies in the midfoot. It does not aid in correction of hindfoot varus or metatarsus adductus.

Surgical technique consists of a dorsal transverse incision over the midfoot region. A curved osteotome is used to fashion the osteotomy. The 1-cm-wide dome osteotomy can be performed through the cuneiforms, cuboid, and base of the fifth metatarsal. The dome shape allows for three-dimensional correction of the deformity and provides optimal bony contact for healing. Steinman pins provide adequate fixation. As with other midfoot osteotomies, a plantar fascial release is often used as an adjunct [26]. Although the procedure is an acceptable alternative to other midfoot osteotomies, it may cause shortening of the foot, and the shape of the osteotomy does not lend itself easily to making bone cuts.

Ilizarov

The Ilizarov method of external fixation is useful for correction of complex foot deformities because of its three-dimensional nature. It may be used with an accompanying midfoot osteotomy for correction of pes cavus. The osteotomy can be safely positioned across the cuboid and navicular or the cuboid and cuneiforms with fluroscopy to form a sufficient surface for bone regeneration [37,49,50].

Advantages of the Ilizarov method include that it is minimally invasive, thus the chance of soft tissue and neurovascular damage is decreased [49]. This method allows for dynamic three-dimensional correction and can simultaneously correct other associated lower extremity deformities [49,51]. The major advantage over internal fixation is that it can be adjusted postoperatively to better obtain the desired correction and position of the foot [49]. Furthermore, its inherent stability allows for early weight bearing and allows for a dynamic repositioning of soft tissue structures to correct a flexible component of the deformity.

Surgical technique may be performed through a single dorsal incision or through the combination of one medial and one lateral incision. Care must be taken to protect the plantar and dorsal neurovascular structures from damage. Our incision placement and dissection is similar to that described by Hamilton and Ford [52]. The medial incision runs from the base of the first metatarsal and proximally to the navicular. The lateral incision is centered over the cuboid. A dorsally based wedge of bone is removed from the midfoot in a similar fashion to the Cole procedure. A V-shaped osteotomy is an acceptable alternative. Surgeons in modern-day Russia often use this V-shaped osteotomy through cancellous bone at the level of the talar neck and calcaneous to promote osseous regeneration. Placement of an Ilizarov frame obviates the need for internal fixation in most cases. Construction of the frame may vary depending on associated conditions. A stable apparatus usually consists of a base frame with at least two proximal rings around the leg [51,53]. The heel frame should consist of crossed smooth wires, half pin in the calcaneous to act as a motor to allow circumferential rotation of the hind foot. Hinges must be placed at the level of the malleoli to allow for the proper rotation. The frame is then completed with a forefoot component at the level of the metatarsals. The patient may begin weight bearing to tolerance as soon as possible. Early weight bearing and dynamic correction make the Ilizarov method of external fixation a viable option for cavus foot deformities.

Miscellaneous midfoot osteotomies

A wide variety of lesser-known midfoot osteotomies have been advocated for the cavus foot. Giannini and associates [54] reviewed one such technique in 39 patients who were treated for idiopathic pes cavus. Treatment consisted of a cuboid osteotomy that was performed in conjunction with a naviculocuneiform

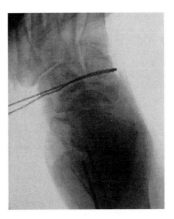

Fig. 11. Placement of giggly saw just before midfoot osteotomy. Care is taken to remain in close contact with bone so as not to injure neurovasculature.

fusion and a plantar fasciotomy. The study reported good or excellent results in 72% of the patients, with success being dependant on patient satisfaction and proper biomechanics of the foot and ankle during postoperative gait analysis [54].

Our institution sometimes performs percutaneus midfoot osteotomies. A giggly saw is used in such cases and provides for an efficient and minimally invasive alternative to a standard osteotomy. A stab incision is placed at the dorsal medial aspect of the midfoot, and special care is taken to perform blunt subperiosteal dissection. The saw is placed through the incision, and care is taken to remain in close contact with the bone so as to remain plantar to all dorsal neurovasculature (Fig. 11). The saw may then exit through a stab incision at the dorsal lateral aspect of the midfoot. Two other stab incisions are created at the plantar medial and plantar lateral aspects, and fluroscopy is then used to ensure proper placement of the saw during the osteotomy (Fig. 12).

Other procedures, such as isolated cuneiform and cuboid osteotomies, can be used as an adjunct. Alone, these procedures have little effect on a cavus

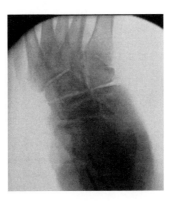

Fig. 12. Midfoot after percutaneous giggly saw osteotomy.

deformity. Cuneiform osteotomy may be useful in aiding in the correction of accompanying metatarsus adductus, whereas a cuboid osteotomy is helpful for residual forefoot abduction that may present with a cavus deformity [55].

Summary

Surgical correction of the cavus foot is a challenging task. It is important to determine the apex of the deformity and to address the entire deformity. It is important to remember that no single procedure can be used exclusively to correct pes cavus. Midfoot osteotomies are an essential component of surgical correction. They can be combined with adjunctive procedures to form an appropriate strategy for the treatment of severe pes cavus.

References

[1] Cole WH. The treatment of claw foot. J Bone Joint Surg 1940;22:895–908.

[2] Japas LM. Surgical treatment of pes cavus by tarsal v-osteotomy. J Bone Joint Surg [Am] 1968;50:927–44.

[3] Berg EE. Chinese foot binding. Orthop Nurs 1995;14:66–8.

[4] Smith TF, Green DR. Pes cavus. In: Banks AS, Downey MS, Martin DE, Miller SJ, editors. McGlamry's comprehensive textbook of foot and ankle surgery. 3rd edition. Philadelphia: Lippincott Williams and Wilkins; 2001. p. 761–98.

[5] Brewerton DA, Sandifer PH, Sweetman DR. Idiopathic pes cavus: an investigation into its etiology. BMJ 1963;1:659–61.

[6] Hsu JD, Mann DC, Imbus CE. Pes cavus. In: Jahss MH, editor. Disorders of the foot and ankle. Philadelphia: WB Saunders; 1991. p. 872–91.

[7] Wapner KL. Pes cavus. In: Myerson MS, editor. Foot and ankle disorders. Philadelphia: WB Saunders; 2000. p. 919–41.

[8] Colon MJ, Whitton KE, Schwartz N. Treatment of pes cavus in a patient with Charcot-Marie-Tooth disease. J Foot Surg 1980;19:41–4.

[9] Fenton CF, McGlamry ED, Perrone M. Severe pes cavus deformity secondary to Charcot-Marie-Tooth disease: a case report. J Am Podiatry Assoc 1982;72:171–5.

[10] Tyrer J. Friedreich's ataxia. In: Vinken PJ, Bruyn GW, DeJong JM, editors. System disorders and atrophies: handbook of clinical neurology, vol. 21. Amsterdam: Elsevier Science; 1975. p. 319–64.

[11] Makin M. The surgical management of Friedreich's ataxia. J Bone Joint Surg [Am] 1953; 35:425–36.

[12] Hansen ST. Cavovarus foot. In: Hurley R, Seigafuse S, Marino D, editors. Functional reconstruction of the foot and ankle. Philadelphia: Lippincott Williams and Wilkins; 2000. p. 209–13.

[13] Ibriham K. Pes cavus. In: Evarts CM, editor. Surgery of the musculoskeletal system. New York: Churchill Livingstone; 1990. p. 4015–34.

[14] Horne G. Pes cavovarus following ankle fracture: a case report. Clin Orthop 1984;184:249–50.

[15] Saunders JT. The etiology and treatment of clubfoot. Arch Surg 1935;30:179–98.

[16] Dwyer FC. The present status of the problem of pes cavus. Clin Orthop 1975;106:254–75.

[17] Schwend RM, Drennan JC. Cavus foot deformity in children. J Am Acad Orthop Surg 2003; 11:201–11.

[18] Mosca VS. The cavus foot. J Pediatr Orthop 2001;21:423–4.

[19] Tynan MC, Klenerman L, Helliweller TR. Investigation of muscle imbalance in the leg and symptomatic forefoot pes cavus in a multidisciplinary study. Foot Ankle 1992;13:489–501.

[20] Olney B. Treatment of the cavus foot Deformity in the pediatric patient with Charcot-Marie-Tooth. Foot Ankle Clin 2000;5(2):305–15.

[21] Coleman SS, Chestnut WJ. A simple test for hindfoot flexibility in the cavovarus foot. Clin Orthop 1977;123:60.

[22] Paulos L, Coleman SS, Samilson KM. Pes cavovarus: review of a surgical approach using selective soft tissue procedures. J Bone Joint Surg [Am] 1980;62:942–53.

[23] Alexander IJ, Johnson KA. Assessment and management of pes cavus and Charcot-Marie-Tooth disease. Clin Orthop 1989;246:273–81.

[24] Jahss MH. Evaluation of the cavus foot for orthopedic treatment. Clin Orthop 1983;181:52–63.

[25] Barenfield PA, Weseley MS, Shea JM. The congenital cavus foot. Clin Orthop 1974;79:119–26.

[26] Wilcox PG, Weiner DS. The Akron midtarsal dome osteotomy in the treatment of rigid pes cavus. J Pediatr Orthop 1985;5(3):333–8.

[27] Jay RM. Cavus deformity. In: Jay RM, Donley S, editors. Pediatric foot and ankle surgery. Philadelphia: WB Saunders; 1999. p. 211–9.

[28] Steinwender W, Linhart WE. High arched forefoot, pes cavus metatarsus congenitus: a case report. Z Orthop Ihre Grenzgeb 1991;129:240–2.

[29] Whitney AK, Green DR. Pseudoequinus. J Am Podiatry Assoc 1982;72:365–71.

[30] Thomas W. On the treatment of talipes cavus. Birmingham Med Rev 1917;34:1–5.

[31] Sherman FC, Westin GW. Plantar release in the correction of deformities of the foot in childhood. J Bone Joint Surg [Am] 1981;63:1382–9.

[32] Steindler A. Operative treatment of pes cavus. Surg Gynecol Obstet 1917;24:612–5.

[33] Steindler A. Stripping of the os calcis. Am J Orthop Surg 1920;2:8–12.

[34] Mann RA. Pes cavus. In: Mann RA, Coughlin MJ, editors. Surgery of the foot and ankle. St. Louis (MO): Mosby; 1993. p. 785–801.

[35] Samilson RL, Dillin W. Cavus, cavovarus, and calcaneovarus: an update. Clin Orthop 1983;177:125–32.

[36] Hansen ST. Tendon transfers and muscle balancing techniques. In: Hurley R, Seigafuse S, Marino D, editors. Functional reconstruction of the foot and ankle. Philadelphia: Lippincott Williams and Wilkins; 2000. p. 433–50.

[37] Holmes JR, Hansen ST. Foot and ankle manifestations of Charcot-Marie-Tooth disease. Foot Ankle 1993;14:476–86.

[38] McGlamry ED, Butlin WE, Ruch JA. Treatment of forefoot equinus by tendon transpositioning. J Am Podiatry Assoc 1975;65:872–88.

[39] Hansen ST. First metatarsal osteotomy for correction of fixed first metatarsal cavus deformity. In: Hurley R, Seigafuse S, Marino D, editors. Functional reconstruction of the foot and ankle. Philadelphia: Lippincott Williams and Wilkins; 2000. p. 391–3.

[40] McElvenny RT, Caldwell GD. A new opereation for correction of cavus foot: fusion of first metatarsocuneiform navicular joints. Clin Orthop 1958;11:85–92.

[41] Perren SM. The biomechanics and biology of internal fixation using plates and nails. Orthopedics 1989;12:21–34.

[42] Jahss MH. Tarsometatarsal truncated-wedge arthrodesis for pes cavus and equinovarus deformity of the fore part of the foot. J Bone Joint Surg [Am] 1980;62:713–22.

[43] Dull JM, DiDomenico LA. Percutaneous displacement calcaneal osteotomy. J Foot Ankle Surg 2004;43(5):336–7.

[44] Dwyer FC. Osteotomy of the calcaneum for pes cavus. J Bone Joint Surg [Br] 1959;41:80–6.

[45] Sullivan RJ, Aronow MS. Different faces of the triple arthrodesis. Foot Ankle Clin 2002;7(1):95–106.

[46] Harley BD. Cole midfoot osteotomy. In: Pediatric foot and ankle surgery. Philadelphia: WB Saunders; 1999. p. 220–4.

[47] Alvik I. Operative treatment of pes cavus. Acta Orthop Scand 1954;23:137–43.

[48] Wulker N, Hurchler C. Cavus foot correction in adults by dorsal closing wedge osteotomy. Foot Ankle Int 2002;23(4):344–7.

[49] Paley D. The correction of complex foot deformities using Ilizarov's distraction osteotomies. Clin Orthop 1993;293:97–111.

[50] Bibbo C, Anderson RB, Davis WH. Complications of midfoot and hindfoot arthrodesis. Clin Orthop 2001;391:45–58.

[51] Ilizarov GA, Shevtsov VI, Shestakov VA, Kuzmin NV. The treatment of foot deformities in adults by the Ilizarov transosseous osteosynthesis. Methodological Recommendation Book. Kurgon, Russia: Kurgon Internal Publication; 1987.

[52] Hamilton GA, Ford LA. External fixation of the foot and ankle elective indications and techniques for external fixation in the midfoot. Clin Podiatr Med Surg 2003;20:45–63.

[53] Kocaoglu M, Eralp L, Atalar AC. Correction of complex foot deformities using Ilizarov external fixator. J Foot Ankle Surg 2002;41(1):30–9.

[54] Giannini S, Ceccarelli F, Benedetti MG, et al. Surgical treatment of adult idiopathic cavus foot with plantar fasciotomy, naviculocuneiform arthrodesis, and cuboid osteotomy: a review of 39 cases. J Bone Joint Surg [Am] 2002;84(2):62–9.

[55] Hall RL. The use of osteotomy to correct foot and ankle deformities. In: Myerson MS, editor. Foot and ankle disorders. Philadelphia: WB Saunders; 2000. p. 1009–10.

ELSEVIER
SAUNDERS

Clin Podiatr Med Surg
22 (2005) 265–276

CLINICS IN
PODIATRIC
MEDICINE AND
SURGERY

The Evans Calcaneal Osteotomy

Brian E. DeYoe, DPM, FACFAS[a],*, Jeremy Wood, DPM[b]

[a]*Podiatric Surgical Associates of North Texas, Baylor University Medical Center,
3600 Gaston Avenue, Wadley Tower, Suite 1056, Dallas, TX 75246, USA*
[b]*Presbyterian Hospital of Greenville, 4215 Joe Ramsey Boulevard, Greenville, TX 75401, USA*

The Evans calcaneal osteotomy is a powerful and proven tool for the correction of the pediatric flexible flatfoot. Originally described by Dr. Evans in 1975 as a wedge osteotomy at the calcaneal neck with tibial cortical graft, the procedure has been modified and its indications have been expanded to correct pediatric and adult flatfoot deformities.

The Evans calcaneal osteotomy has developed into the premier procedure for lateral column lengthening. There are, however, pitfalls and contraindications associated with the procedure. Proper patient selection is imperative to a successful outcome with this procedure.

Preoperative criteria

The first and foremost indication is flexibility. Any amount of rigidity can dramatically reduce the amount of correction obtained [1]. The foot should also exhibit calcaneal valgus, forefoot abduction, and peritalar subluxation. The patient should also exhibit calcaneal maturity sufficient for osteotomy and graft interposition. This most commonly occurs at age 8, but can vary by as many as 2 years (Fig. 1).

Underlying tarsal coalition is not an absolute contraindication for this procedure. The author has performed the procedure on patients with calcaneo-navicular coalitions. Success can be achieved, provided that resection of the osseous bar allows the foot to become flexible. If the foot remains semirigid to rigid because of underlying soft tissue adaptation or arthrosis, an Evans calcaneal

---

* Corresponding author.
E-mail address: bdeyoe@northtexaspodiatry.com (B.E. DeYoe).

0891-8422/05/$ – see front matter © 2005 Elsevier Inc. All rights reserved.
doi:10.1016/j.cpm.2004.10.002   *podiatric.theclinics.com*

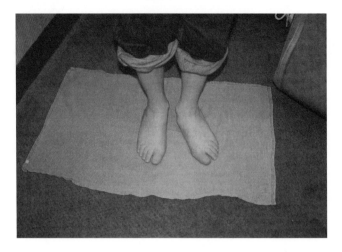

Fig. 1. A 10-year-old patient showing the correction obtained with the Evans calcaneal osteotomy on the right foot in comparison to the nonoperative foot on the left.

osteotomy is contraindicated. Talocalcaneal coalitions are generally a contra-indication, especially if adaptive changes of the posterior facet have occurred. A talonavicular coalition is an absolute contraindication for the Evans procedure [2].

Hindfoot arthrosis is also a contraindication. If the affected joint is mobile and easily reducible then an Evans calcaneal osteotomy can be performed. There has been considerable discussion in the literature that the Evans procedure is contraindicated if a patient exhibits calcanealcuboid arthrosis. Cooper et al [3] performed a study on eight cadaver specimens that revealed an increase in pressure at the calcanealcuboid (c-c) joint after an Evans lateral column-lengthening procedure. This increase in pressure is believed to cause arthrosis of the calcanealcuboid joint [4]. The major flaw of this study is that it involves cadaver specimens, which does not allow for evaluation of soft tissue adaptation, or long-term follow-up. Momberger et al [5] studies revealed "the change in pressure from the flatfoot to the corrected foot was not significant, and in some cases peak pressures in the corrected foot were actually lower than in the flatfoot." This is consistent with the author's belief that c-c joint pressures decrease postprocedure. The belief is that by restoring the c-c joint to a proper rectus alignment, joint pressures decrease (and increase with malignment). The Evans procedure performed on a semirigid-to-rigid deformity can increase joint pressure as a result of lack of correction and impaction of the joint. The authors have never seen athrosis of the c-c joint occur post-Evans procedure.

Metatarsus adductus is another contraindication commonly reported with the Evans procedure. The surgeon must evaluate the severity and surgical options for the patient. The Evans procedure can be performed on patients with mild-to-moderate deformity with only minimal increase to their metatarsus adductus angle. In a study by Brim and Hecker [6], it was concluded that the metatarsus angle increased by 1.5 degrees. The surgeon should be cautious in severe deformities where even small increases in deformity can have profound effect. The Evans procedure can be performed in patients with severe deformity provided they exhibit increased c-c joint angle and peritalar subluxation. Underlying metatarsus adductus can then be surgically addressed.

Physical examination

The Evans procedure requires flexibility to correct the underlying deformity. When examining the patient preoperatively the surgeon should be able to reduce the deformity easily. The heel should be easily reduced from its valgus position, as well as forefoot abduction [7]. This allows for the rearticulation of the talonavicular joint, thereby reducing the deformity. Any amount of rigidity should rule out underlying arthrosis or tarsal coalition.

The practitioner should also check for underlying equinus by having the patient extend the leg fully, placing the heel in neutral position. The foot is then dorsiflexed and evaluated. Failure to place the heel in neutral position upon evaluation will result in a false amount of available dorsiflexion. This examination is important because post-Evans procedure the patient will lose 5 to 15 degrees of available dorsiflexion depending on the amount of heel valgus.

The strength of posterior tibial tendon and muscle group should also be evaluated. This is evaluated by having the patient plantarflex and invert the foot. They are instructed to resist the surgeon who is trying to forcefully evert and dorsiflex the foot. Another way to examine the posterior tibial muscle group is to have the patient perform a single-heel raise test. The patient faces the wall with the contralateral leg flexed at the knee. The patient then performs a heel raise. The heel should invert during the first two-thirds of plantarflexion. If the heel remains in valgus, the posterior tibial muscle group is not functioning properly. Further evaluation for tear or attenuation of the posterior tibial tendon, hypertrophy of the navicular tuberosity, or os navicularis is needed. An adjunctive procedure should be performed in conjunction with the Evans calcaneal osteotomy to address posterior tibial tendon dysfunction [8–10].

Radiographic examination

Weight-bearing radiographs are essential in evaluating a patient's flexible flatfoot deformity, as there are dramatic changes between the weight bearing and non–weight-bearing foot. Indicators of a flexible flatfoot on a lateral plain view are an anterior break in the cyma line, increased talar declination, decreased calcaneal inclination, superimposition of the metatarsals, and a decreased declination of the first metatarsal (Fig. 2).

The dorsoplantar (AP) view demonstrates an increased talocalcaneal angle (Kite's angle), decreased talonavicular articulation (often less than 50%), forefoot abductus, and an incongruous calcanealcuboid joint with cuboid abductus (Fig. 3).

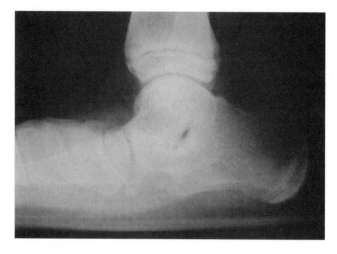

Fig. 2. Lateral view exhibiting anterior break in the cyma line, increased talar declination, and decreased calcaneal inclination.

Other diagnostic imaging can be helpful in ruling out tarsal coalitions, such as a CT scan. Magnetic resonance imaging can be useful in evaluating tendon tears and attenuations, as well as synchondrotic and syndesmotic tarsal coalitions in children and juveniles (Fig. 4).

The average radiographic improvement upon post-Evan's procedure in the lateral talocalcaneal angle was 6.4 degrees, and the anteroposterior talocalcaneal

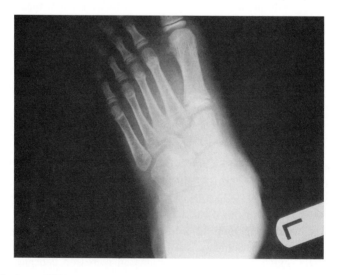

Fig. 3. AP view exhibiting increased Kite's angle, decreased talonavicular articulation, and forefoot abduction.

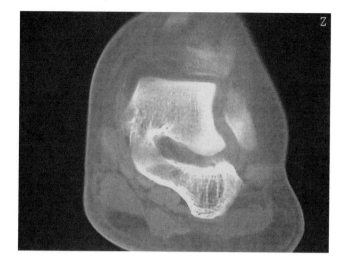

Fig. 4. CT axial view exhibiting osseous coalition of the middle facet of the subtalar joint.

angle improved on average 15.9 degrees. The articulation between the talus and the navicular also increased significantly [11,12].

Procedure

The incision is started 1 cm distal to the lateral malleolus and carried to the calcaneocuboid (c-c) joint. This provides excellent exposure while avoiding injury to the intermediate dorsal cutaneous and sural nerve (Fig. 5).

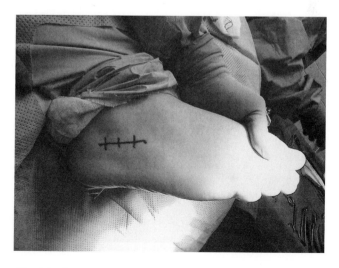

Fig. 5. Preferred incisional approach for the Evans calcaneal osteotomy.

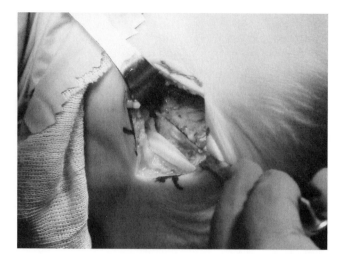

Fig. 6. Osteotomy placed at the base of the anterior superior process of the calcaneus where it meets the sinus tarsi.

Dissection is performed to the extensor digitorum brevis (EDB) and peroneal tendons. An incision is placed between the two structures, and the EDB is reflected dorsally and the peroneal tendons plantarly. Care is taken to protect the soft tissue attachments at the level of the c-c joint. Failure to do so can result in avascular necrosis or subluxation of the distal fragment of the calcaneus.

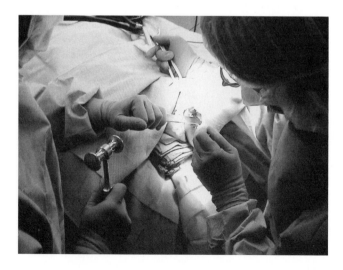

Fig. 7. Author using an osteotome to finish osteotomy and loosen soft tissue adhesions.

The osteotomy is placed 1 cm to 1.5 cm proximal to the c-c joint. This is usually where the anterior superior portion of the calcaneus meets the floor of the sinus tarsi. The authors use this as there anatomical landmark for the site of the osteotomy. Making the osteotomy at this level allows for the anterior and middle facet to be bisected (Fig. 6).

Before the osteotomy is performed a .062 k-wire is passed percutaneously from distal to proximal across the c-c joint as temporary fixation to prevent subluxation of the distal fragment of the calcaneus. The osteotomy is placed from lateral to medial in a through-and-through fashion. The authors usually begin the osteotomy with a saw and finish with an osteotome. This lessens the possibility of damage to medial structures and allows the surgeon to use the osteotome as a lever arm in loosening the osseous structures from its soft tissue adhesions. The soft tissue structures are freed from their osseous adhesions by moving the osteotome from side to side within the osteotomy (Fig. 7).

The osteotomy is distracted using a smooth straight laminar spreader or minidistractor to the amount of correction desired. This is determined through intraoperative fluroscopy with the foot in a loaded position. The surgeon should distract the osteotomy until the talonavicular joint is rearticulated and the lateral column is straight (Fig. 8).

The amount of distraction necessary to correct the deformity determines the size of bone graft needed. Autograft is not necessary because the calcaneus is vascular and has mostly cancellous bone. There are many viable options in selecting bone grafting material, including iliac crest, patella, and femoral head

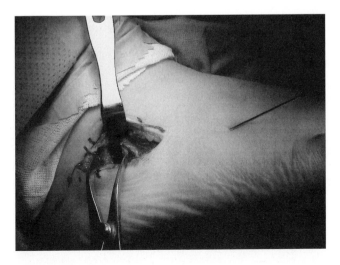

Fig. 8. Osteotomy is distracted to the desired amount of correction. Also note placement of percutaneous k-wire to prevent c-c joint subluxation.

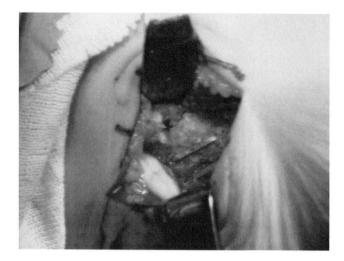

Fig. 9. Graft placement with staple fixation.

[13,14]. The authors prefer alloimplant calcaneal cross-section grafts, which are identical to the calcaneus at the site of osteotomy. Calcaneal cross-section grafts provide structural cortical support while promoting cancellous proliferation. Because it is an allograft, there is no donor site morbidity and surgical time, which would be spent obtaining an autogenous graft, is decreased.

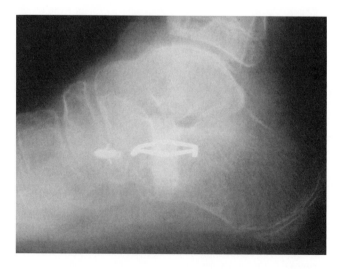

Fig. 10. Lateral view showing early incorporation of graft at 6 weeks.

Once the graft is placed, the osteotomy is fixated, though not as described originally by Dr. Evans. The authors believe that the osteotomy should be fixated to avoid loss of correction during graft incorporation and to prevent dislocation of the graft. They also believe that screw and k-wire fixation are inadequate; though they prevent dislocation of the graft, they do little to prevent loss of correction during graft incorporation. For this reason, staple or plate fixation is recommended. Both procedures prevent graft dislocation and loss of correction during graft incorporation by maintaining length (Fig. 9) [15].

Postoperative care

The patient is placed initially non-weight bearing in a well-padded sugar tong splint for 2 weeks until the sutures are removed. A short-leg non–weight-bearing cast is then applied for 6 weeks or until the graft shows early incorporation on radiograph (Fig. 10).

The patient is then placed weight bearing in a fracture walker boot or short-leg cast for 4 to 6 weeks. The patient is then gradually placed weight bearing in athletic shoes. The patient is to refrain from athletic or high-impact activities for 6 months (Fig. 11).

Complications

The overall complication rate with the Evans calcaneal osteotomy is low, but as with all surgeries, complications can occur. Some of the most common

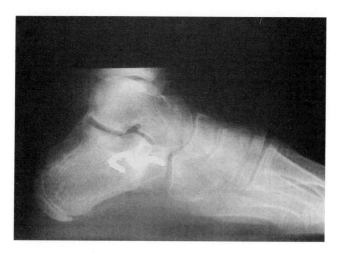

Fig. 11. Lateral view showing complete incorporation of graft at 6 months.

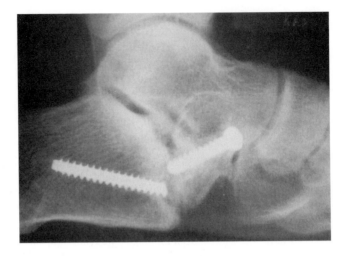

Fig. 12. Lateral view showing nonunion at 8 months after patient was allowed full, unprotected weight bearing at 6 weeks.

complications associated with the procedure include delayed union, nonunion, and malunion [16]. Lesser complications (with potentially increased morbidity) include avascular necrosis, subluxation of the distal fragment of the calcaneus, nerve injury, and c-c joint impaction. Although rare, stress fractures of the fifth metatarsal have been reported (Figs. 12 and 13) [17].

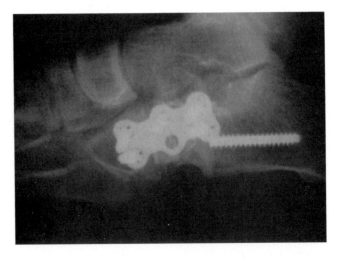

Fig. 13. Revision of nonunion with c-c joint arthrodesis and interpositional autogenous iliac crest graft.

Proper preoperative planning, which includes the following, can prevent most complications:

1. The patient must have a flexible flatfoot preoperatively. The more rigid the foot, the less likely a successful outcome is possible.
2. Proper graft selection is important. Cortical bone wedges are often used, which can slow osseous proliferation and lead to a delayed union or nonunion. The ideal graft would contain an outer cortical bone for structural support and an inner cancellous bone to promote proliferation. A calcanceal cross-section allograft works well to meet both these needs.
3. Nerve damage of the sural or dorsal intermediate nerves can be avoided by careful dissection and incision placement.
4. The risk of avascular necrosis of the distal fragment of the calcaneus is decreased by minimizing dissection at the c-c joint.
5. Subluxation of the distal fragment of the calcaneus is lessened by performing minimal dissection at the c-c joint and by using staple or plate fixation across the graft site.

Discussion

The foot and ankle surgeon has many surgical options when addressing the flexible flatfoot. The Evans calcaneal osteotomy is able to correct the most severe disorders from the pediatric patient to the young adult and can repair underlying deformity without joint arthrodesis or extraarticular implant. Combined with its low incedence of complication and proven long-term track record, it should remain in the foot and ankle surgeon's arsenal.

References

[1] Mahan KT, McGlamry ED. Evans calcaneal osteotomy for pes valgus deformity. Clin Pod Med Surg 1987;4(4):806–11.
[2] Giannini S, Ceccarelli F, Vannini F, et al. Operative treatment of flatfoot with talocalcaneal coalition. Clin Orthop 2003;1(411):178–87.
[3] Cooper PS, Nowak MD, Shaer J. Calcanealcubiod joint pressures with lateral column lengthening (Evans) procedure. Foot Ankle Int 1997;18(4):199–205.
[4] Mosier-LaClair S, Pomeroy G, Manoli A. Operative treatment of the difficult stage 2 adult acquired flatfoot deformity. Foot Ankle Clin 2001;6(1):95–119.
[5] Momberger N, Morgan JM, et al. Calcanealcuboid joint pressure after lateral column lengthening in a cadaveric planovalgus deformity model. Foot Ankle Int 2000;21(9):730–5.
[6] Brim SP, Hecker R. The Evans calcaneal osteotomy. J Foot Ankle Surg 1994;33(1):2–5.
[7] Dollard MD, et al. The Evans calcaneal osteotomy for correction of flexible flatfoot syndrome. J Foot Surg 1984;23(4):291–301.
[8] El-Tayeby HM. The severe flexible flatfoot. J Foot Ankle Surg 1999;38(1):41–9.
[9] Lombardi CM, et al. Talonavicular joint arthrodesis and Evans calcaneal osteotomy treatment of posterior tibial tendon dysfunction. J Foot Ankle Surg 1999;38(2):116–22.

[10] Bruyn JM, Cerniglia MW, Chaney DM. Combination of Evans calcaneal osteotomy and STA-Peg arthroreisis for correction of the severe pes valgo planus deformity. J Foot Ankle Surg 1999;38(5):339–46.

[11] Sangeorzan BJ, Mosca V, Hansen Jr ST. Effect of calcaneal lengthening on relationships among the hindfoot, midfoot, and forefoot. Foot Ankle 1993;14(3):136–41.

[12] Viegas GV. Reconstruction of the pediatric flexible planovalgus foot by using and Evans calcaneal osteotomy and augmentative medial split tibialis anterior tendon transfer. J Foot Ankle Surg 2003;42(4):199–207.

[13] Mahan KT, Hillstrom HJ. Bone grafting in foot and ankle surgery. J Am Pod Med Assoc 1998;88(3):109–18.

[14] Mosca VS. Calcaneal lengthening for valgus deformity of the hindfoot. J Bone Joint Surg [Am] 1995;77(4):500–12.

[15] Hansen S. Progressive symptomatic flat foot. In: Hansen ST, editor. Reconstruction of the foot and ankle. Philadelphia: Lippincott, Williams and Wilkins; 2000. p. 195–207.

[16] Thomas RL, et al. Preliminary results comparing two methods of lateral column lengthening. Foot Ankle Int 2001;22(2):107–19.

[17] Davitt JS, Morgan JM. Stress fracture of the fifth metatarsal after Evans calcaneal osteotomy. Foot Ankle Int 1998;19(10):710–2.

ELSEVIER
SAUNDERS

Clin Podiatr Med Surg
22 (2005) 277–289

CLINICS IN
PODIATRIC
MEDICINE AND
SURGERY

Posterior Calcaneal Displacement Osteotomy for the Adult Acquired Flatfoot

Michael S. Lee, DPM, FACFAS

Central Iowa Orthopaedics, 1601 NW 114th Street, Suite 142, Des Moines, IA 50325, USA

Posterior tibial tendon dysfunction (PTTD) resulting in the adult acquired flatfoot is a common condition challenging the foot and ankle surgeon. The condition is progressive in nature and may present as localized tenosynovitis, complete rupture of the tendon with a supple flatfoot, or as a nonreducible flatfoot with ankle involvement. Surgical treatment of this condition is dictated by the severity and progression of the deformity. Despite its prevalence, controversies surround the surgical management of this condition, particularly when the adult acquired flatfoot remains reducible.

Numerous classifications have been advocated [1–4]. Johnson and Strom's [1] classification is the most widely accepted classification system for posterior tibial tendon dysfunction as it describes the status of the posterior tibial tendon, as well as rigidity (or reducibility) of the rearfoot (Table 1). Stage I demonstrates tenosynovitis with normal tendon length and minimal to no structural deformity. A stage II deformity represents a supple flatfoot with attenuation or rupture of the posterior tibial tendon. Early in stage II, the pain is generally medial, whereas in more progressive stage II deformities the symptoms will often be more lateral. Stage III deformities are characterized by a rigid (nonreducible) flatfoot [1]. Stage IV deformities, as modified by Myerson [4]; show a rigid flatfoot with ankle involvement.

Tenosynovitis of the posterior tibial tendon was first recognized in 1936, but the dysfunction of a partially torn posterior tibial tendon was not recognized until 1953 [5,6]. Early surgical management of the inflamed tendon centered on debridement of the tendon with or without transfer of one of the flexor tendons [7–9]. These procedures were noted to provide adequate symptomatic relief of the condition but virtually no correction of the flatfoot deformity [9].

Surgical reconstruction of the stage II deformity has subsequently focused on osseous correction of the deformity. Isolated subtalar, calcaneocuboid, and

Table 1
Johnson and Strom classification system for posterior tibial tendon dysfunction with adult acquired flatfoot

Stage	Clinical findings	Radiographic findings	Posterior tibial tendon pathology
I	Medial swelling and pain. No loss of arch height. Normal hindfoot range of motion.	Typically no radiographic changes.	Tenosynovitis with no to minimal attenuation.
II	Early medial swelling and pain along the course of the tendon, normal motion; late lateral pain with some reduction of motion	Collapse of medial arch. Increase angular deformity including talo-first metatarsal angles (AP and lateral), cuboid abduction angle, and peritalar subluxation.	Attenuation or complete rupture of posterior tibial tendon.
III	Rigid flatfoot with nonreducible subtalar joint. Pain laterally, sinus tarsi and subfibular.	Radiographic angles as in stage II. Hindfoot arthrosis and degenerative changes.	Same as stage II.
IV	Same as stage III with the addition of ankle pain and subluxation.	Same as stage III with ankle valgus and degeneration.	Same as stage II and III.

Data from Johnson KA, Strom DE. Tibialis posterior tendon dysfunction. Clin Orthop 1989 Feb; (239):196–206; and Myerson MS. Adult acquired flatfoot deformity. J Bone Joint Surg [Am] 1996;78:780.

talonavicular joint arthrodesis as well as double arthrodesis have also been recommended for stage II deformities [10–16]. These isolated fusions of the hindfoot have generally provided excellent correction. However, the restriction of hindfoot motion after isolated fusion has been documented and may result in long-term arthrosis [17,18].

Most of the controversy surrounding surgical management of PTTD is centered on the management of Johnson and Strom stage II deformities [1]. Gleich [19] first described the use of a calcaneal osteotomy to reestablish calcaneal inclination. Koutsogiannis [20] used an osteotomy through the posterior calcaneus to correct the mobile flatfoot. The posterior calcaneal displacement osteotomy (PCDO) with flexor digitorum longus (FDL) tendon transfer for the adult acquired flatfoot is one of many accepted approaches to this complicated condition. Indications, contraindications, and procedure technique are discussed.

Indications

Posterior calcaneal displacement osteotomy with FDL transfer is indicated for the stage II posterior tibial tendon dysfunction. Individuals with this condition demonstrate varying degrees of medial column arch collapse, forefoot abduction, and hindfoot valgus. The deformity should be supple with a reducible subtalar joint. Additionally, there should be no evidence of forefoot varus or midtarsal joint arthrosis. In the presence of a supple hindfoot with a fixed forefoot varus, ancillary medial column procedures may be warranted to reduce the forefoot varus deformity [21].

Contraindications

The PCDO is contraindicated in individuals with stage III or IV posterior tibial tendon dysfunction. The hindfoot arthrosis and rigid nature of these deformities prevents correction with reconstructive osteotomies. Additionally, comorbid conditions, including obesity, diabetes, history of smoking, and activity limitations, may serve as relative contraindications [22].

Operative technique

The patient is positioned on the operative table in the supine position with a thigh tourniquet under general or spinal anesthesia. Though the calcaneal osteotomy is more easily performed with the patient in the lateral position, the author prefers the supine position to limit the need for repositioning the patient for completion of medial tendon transfers or medial column arthrodesis procedures. The supine position also makes it easier to obtain critical fluoroscopic radiographs.

The posterior muscle group contracture is addressed initially. Tendo-Achilles lengthening or a gastrocnemius recession is completed according to clinical exam and surgeon preference. Both procedures are easily completed with the patient in the supine position. When a tendo-Achilles lengthening is selected, a percutaneus, triple-hemi-section technique is used. This is completed with the extremity elevated by an assistant. Three stab incisions are created directly overlying the Achilles tendon, approximately 2 cm apart, and beginning 2 cm proximal to the superior border of the calcaneus. The Achilles is sectioned from midline to lateral in the proximal and distal incisions and from midline to medial in the central incision. Dorsiflexion of the ankle with the subtalar joint in neutral position allows the Achilles tendon to lengthen upon itself. Care should be taken not to overlengthen or rupture the tendon during dorsiflexion.

The gastrocnemius recession is the author's preferred technique because it preserves strength, decreases the risk of Achilles rupture, and limits rehabilitation required postoperatively. This procedure is also easily completed with the patient in the supine position. The heel is placed on a stack of towels to elevate the gastrocnemius muscle belly from the table. A medial approach is created at the myotendinous junction of the medial gastrocnemius muscle belly (Fig. 1A). Dissection is carried deep to the crural fascia; a linear incision through the crural fascia then exposes the deep fatty tissue layer overlying the gastrocnemius

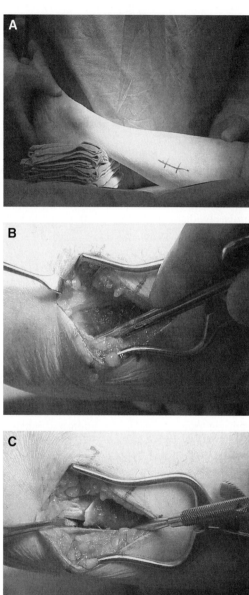

Fig. 1. (*A*) Extremity placement and incisional approach for a supine, medial approach gastrocnemius recession; (*B*) identification of the crural fascia and the gastrocnemius aponeurosis; (*C*) transsection of the gastrocnemius aponeurosis with identification of the deeper soleal aponeurosis.

aponeurosis (Fig. 1B). The aponeurosis is then identified, and the soft tissues are elevated off the aponeurosis from medial to lateral using blunt dissection. Care must be taken to ensure that the sural nerve and lesser saphenous vein are elevated within the soft tissues off the aponeurosis as they cross near the midline of the aponeurosis. These vital structures are retracted off the aponeurosis using a freer elevator. The medial border of the aponeurosis is then identified, and sectioning of the gastrocnemius aponeurosis is performed from medial to lateral (Fig. 1C). Care should be taken to leave the deeper soleus aponeurosis intact. The lateral portion of the gastrocnemius aponeurosis is often transected using a somewhat blind technique. Dorsiflexion of the ankle will demonstrate adequate lengthening of the gastrocnemius aponeurosis. Deep closure of the crural fascia is performed with an interrupted absorbable stitch; skin closure is according to surgeon preference.

Attention is then directed to the lateral calcaneal region. A large bump under the ipsilateral hip will facilitate internal rotation of the hip and exposure to the lateral heel. The incision is placed parallel to the peroneal tendons, just posterior and inferior to the course of the sural nerve (Fig. 2). The incision should extend from just anterior to the Achilles tendon and superior to the calcaneus to a point distal and inferior to the weight-bearing surface of the calcaneus. Dissection is carried directly to bone, and the periosteum is incised in the same plane as the skin incision. Subperiosteal dissection is completed to visualize the superior and inferior borders of the calcaneus (Fig. 3). Care should be taken to limit excessive retraction of the skin margins as the skin closure may become somewhat tenuous after translation of the posterior calcaneal segment.

A through-and-through osteotomy is then completed in the same plane as the skin and periosteal incisions, and should be approximately 45° to the weight-bearing surface. Care should be taken superiorly to protect the Achilles tendon, and inferiorly to protect the plantar structures. One must also use caution when exiting the medial cortex as the medial neurovascular structures may be at risk.

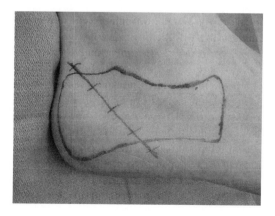

Fig. 2. Incision placement running parallel to the peroneal tendons; posterior and inferior to the sural nerve.

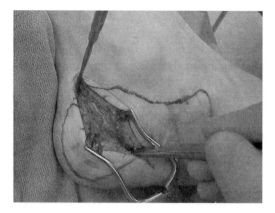

Fig. 3. Subperiosteal dissection with identification of the superior and inferior borders of the calcaneus.

A feathering type of motion is used to transect the medial calcaneal cortex. A toothless lamina spreader is then inserted into the osteotomy; opening and closing the lamina spreader several times will help to stretch the medial periosteum and facilitate translation of the posterior segment (Fig. 4).

The posterior segment of the calcaneus is then translated medially 10 to 15 mm and temporarily fixated with a 0.062-inch Kirschner wire (Fig. 5A). Adequate correction is confirmed with a calcaneal axial view using flouroscopy (Fig. 5B). Caution should be taken to prevent overcorrection as this may cause the posterior segment to "teeter" into a varus malalignment. Permanent fixation is then achieved using one or two large-diameter cannulated screws placed from posterior to anterior across the osteotomy (Fig. 6). Fixation placement is confirmed using flouroscopy. Care should be taken to prevent subtalar joint invasion with the final fixation.

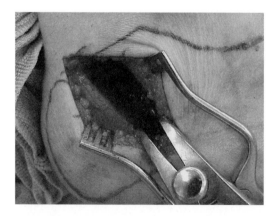

Fig. 4. Lamina spreader within the posterior calcaneal displacement osteotomy being used to manipulate the medial periosteal structures to facilitate medial translation of the posterior segment.

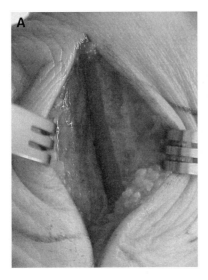
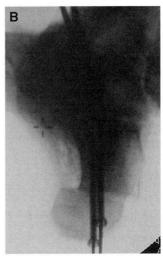

Fig. 5. (*A*) 1-cm correction after medialization of the posterior segment; (*B*) calcaneal axial view demonstrating appropriate medial translation of the posterior segment and internal fixation placement.

Adjunctive medial procedures are then completed after removal of the ipsilateral hip bump to facilitate external rotation of the hip. Typically, a flexor digitorum longus tendon transfer is completed with debridement and repair of the posterior tibial tendon. The tendon transfer is completed according to surgeon preference. The author most typically completes a weave-type transfer of the FDL into the posterior tibial tendon (Fig. 7). The distal stump of the FDL is passed through a drill hole in the navicular tuberosity. The spring ligament may also be repaired. Medial column fusions may be used adjunctively.

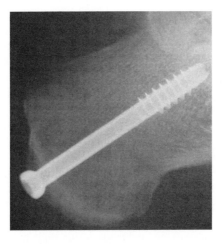

Fig. 6. Lateral view demonstrating proper fixation placement with a large cannulated screw.

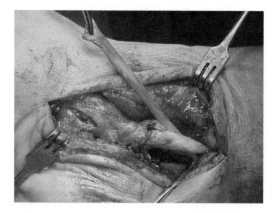

Fig. 7. FDL tendon weave transfer to the posterior tibial tendon.

The patient is placed in a well-padded posterior splint. Sutures are removed at 10 to 14 days and the extremity is placed in a below-the-knee fiberglass cast for 3 to 4 weeks. Partial weight bearing is allowed 5 weeks postoperatively in the fiberglass cast and full weight bearing is initiated in a walking boot 6 weeks postoperatively. The patient is progressed to sneakers with a lightweight ankle brace at 9 weeks. Physical therapy is used for complete rehabilitation.

Discussion

Controversy in the management of stage II PTTD deformities surrounds the use of isolated hindfoot arthrodesis, subtalar arthroeresis, and reconstructive osteotomies. A great deal of variation amongst foot and ankle surgeons exists in the management of stage II deformities [23]. Some of this variation may be dependent on the surgeon's region of practice and training experience.

Isolated subtalar joint arthrodesis has been used for the correction of stage II PTTD [14,24–28]. In most cases, FDL tendon transfer is used to antagonize the peroneus brevis tendon pull and prevent pronation through the midtarsal joint. Union rates with isolated subtalar joint arthrodesis are high throughout the literature [29]. However, simulated subtalar joint arthrodesis was noted to restrict talonavicular joint motion by as much as 74% [17]. This limitation of midtarsal joint motion after subtalar arthrodesis may result in progressive degenerative changes of the midtarsal joint [30].

The talonavicular arthrodesis has many advantages, including excellent correction of the medial longitudinal arch, correction of hindfoot valgus, and the exclusion of FDL tendon transfer [10,11,31]. Limitation of subtalar joint motion to less than 8° after talonavicular arthrodesis has affected the procedures acceptance [17]. Because of this reduction in hindfoot motion, the procedure is more often indicated in low-demand patients with significant stage II deformity.

Unlike isolated subtalar and talonavicular joint arthrodeses, a sufficient amount of motion may be maintained with calcaneocuboid joint distraction arthrodesis [17,18]. Subtalar joint range of motion ranges from 50% to 80% of normal after calcaneocuboid joint distraction arthrodesis [18]. Autogenous bone grafting is necessary to provide length in the lateral column and correction of deformity. The increased morbidity with bone grafting and risk of nonunion are considerable disadvantages to the procedure.

Several reconstructive osteotomies have been described for the adult-acquired flatfoot, including most notably the Evans calcaneal osteotomy and posterior calcaneal displacement osteotomy. Generally, the advantage of reconstructive osteotomies over isolated arthrodesis is the ability to maintain hindfoot motion. Though reconstructive osteotomies may limit or alter hindfoot motion, they are considered to be less limiting than isolated hindfoot arthrodeses.

The Evans calcaneal osteotomy provides correction of the adult flatfoot by reducing forefoot abduction, increasing first ray plantarflexion, and reducing hindfoot valgus [32,33]. Concerns regarding increased calcaneocuboid joint pressures has affected wide range acceptance in adults [34,35]. Combining PCDO with Evans calcaneal osteotomy has also been used, especially in the presence of significant flatfoot deformity or when significant forefoot abduction is noted [36–40].

Koutsogiannis [20] is typically given credit for describing today's medializing osteotomy of the posterior segment of the calcaneus. Though many other calcaneal osteotomies have been described for flatfoot correction, medializing the posterior segment of the calcaneal body remains one of the most often used [19,22,41–48]. The rationale for this procedure is based on its ability to re-establish the Achilles tendon as a heel invertor as the insertion of the Achilles is shifted from lateral to medial of the subtalar joint axis [43,45,49,50]. Hindfoot supination is also increased as ground reactive forces occur medial to the subtalar joint axis of motion [45].

The posterior calcaneal displacement osteotomy has also been reported to reduce a flexible forefoot varus (supinatus) [20,21,51]. The PCDO was once theorized to recreate the medial longitudinal arch by tightening the plantar fascia and increasing the windlass mechanism [52]. More recent studies have disproved this theory and demonstrate that the plantar fascia is actually relaxed after PCDO [53,54].

The PCDO is indicated for the stage II PTTD flatfoot. The presence of midtarsal joint arthrosis or a fixed forefoot varus precludes its use. The osteotomy has often been used in conjunction with a FDL tendon transfer and posterior muscle group lengthening [22,43–47]. It has been demonstrated that PCDO with FDL tendon transfer performs subjectively better than PCDO without FDL tendon transfer [44]. The PCDO will offset the inherent weakness found in isolated FDL tendon transfers by reducing the heel valgus and its antagonistic pronatory forces [9,46].

Radiographic evaluations of the PCDO have demonstrated its ability to correct the talo-first metatarsal angle on the anteroposterior (AP) radiograph as much as 11° to 12° [44,46]. Talo-first metatarsal angle correction on lateral radiographs was noted to have similar effects on correction, with greater than 13° correction noted [44,46]. Additionally, the PCDO causes a reduction in talar head uncovering, limiting talar pronation and peritalar subluxation [46]. These radiographic studies demonstrate the effectiveness of the PCDO in correcting moderate changes in the medial longitudinal arch and forefoot abduction seen with the adult-acquired flatfoot.

Postoperative subjective outcomes with PCDO have been noted to be less favorable when preoperative talo-first metatarsal angles on both the AP and lateral radiographs were greater than 25° [44]. These findings have demonstrated the procedure's inability to adequately correct more severe deformities. Evaluation of the talo-first metatarsal angles on the AP and lateral weight-bearing radiographs is critical to proper procedure selection. In cases with elevated angles, patients may benefit from double calcaneal osteotomy or isolated hindfoot arthrodesis.

A disadvantage of the PCDO is its inability to correct significant forefoot abduction in the adult-acquired flatfoot. Patients with significant forefoot abduction as noted by increased AP talo-first metatarsal and cuboid abduction angles may be treated with double calcaneal osteotomy or calcaneocuboid distraction arthrodesis. Additionally, PCDO has been shown to alter tibiotalar joint mechanics and distribution of contact stresses, which may result in long-term ankle joint degenerative changes [55–57].

The long-term outcomes of PCDO are not yet known. Several intermediate-term studies with greater than 30 months mean follow-up have demonstrated favorable subjective outcomes [58–60]. Patients were noted to have improved functional results and demonstrate the ability to complete single heel rise test postoperatively [58–60]. In one study, patients noted a prolonged period of steady improvement in symptoms and function [58].

Complications associated with the PCDO are rare. Patients may experience sural neuritis or peroneal tendonitis associated with the lateral incision [44]. Care should be taken to place the lateral incision parallel to the course of the peroneal tendons but far enough posterior to avoid the sural nerve. Limiting soft tissue dissection to subperiosteal dissection will also limit the occurrence of sural nerve entrapment and neuritis. The through-and-through osteotomy has been shown to put several of the medial neurovascular structures at risk for injury, including the medial and lateral plantar nerves, the medial calcaneal nerve, and the medial vascular structures.

Delayed or nonunions are extremely rare with this type of osteotomy [22]. The highly vascular, cancellous bone in the posterior calcaneus limits concerns for proper bone healing. Adequate countersinking of the posterior screw head can limit posterior irritation. If the screw head remains prominent, patients may complain of irritation once weight bearing in normal shoe gear is initiated. In some cases, scar tissue along the posterior heel may cause transient problems. Patients may perceive this to be the screws. A silicone heel cup will often provide relief as the scar tissue is reorganized. The lateral (and less often medial) cortical shelf may also cause shoe gear irritation, especially early in the recovery process.

Rearfoot arthrosis may be noted postoperatively. The osteotomy alters rearfoot and ankle mechanics, but in many cases the arthrosis seen may represent a continuum of early arthrosis present preoperatively [22]. Undercorrection, with less than 10 mm medial translation may result in residual deformity and less favorable subjective outcomes [44]. Gaining adequate medialization of the posterior segment is often limited by the thick medial periosteum. Stretching the medial soft tissues with a lamina spreader will improve the medial shift.

Summary

The posterior calcaneal displacement osteotomy with FDL transfer remains a viable option for the stage II PTTD flatfoot with mild to moderate radiographic deformity. Proper patient selection and adequate medialization of the posterior segment greatly affects outcomes. Additionally, combining PCDO with the flexor digitorum transfer positively affects results. Complications, though rare, may include sural neuritis, peroneal tendonitis, undercorrection, and peritalar arthrosis.

References

[1] Johnson KA, Strom DE. Tibialis posterior tendon dysfunction. Clin Orthop 1989 Feb;(239): 196–206.
[2] Mueller TJ. Acquired flatfoot secondary to tibialis posterior dysfunction: biomechanical aspects. J Foot Surg 1991;30(1):2–11.
[3] Conti SF, Michelson J, Jahss MH. Clinical significance of magnetic resonance imaging in preoperative planning for reconstruction of posterior tibial tendon ruptures. Foot Ankle 1992; 13:208–14.
[4] Myerson MS. Adult acquired flatfoot deformity. J Bone Joint Surg [Am] 1996;78:780.
[5] Key JA. Partial rupture of the tendon of the posterior tibial muscle. J Bone Joint Surg 1953;35:1006–8.
[6] Kulowski J. Tendovaginitis (tenosynovitis). J Miss State Med Assoc 1936;33:135.
[7] Johnson KA. Tibialis posterior tendon rupture. Clin Orthop 1983 Jul–Aug;(177):140–7.
[8] Jahss MH. Spontaneous rupture of the tibialis posterior tendon: clinical findings, tenographic studies, and a new technique of repair. Foot Ankle 1982;3(3):158–66.
[9] Mann RA, Thompson FM. Rupture of the posterior tibial tendon causing flat foot. Surgical treatment. J Bone Joint Surg [Am] 1985;67(4):556–61.
[10] Harper MC, Tisdel CL. Talonavicular arthrodesis for the painful adult acquired flatfoot. Foot Ankle Int 1996;17(11):658–61.
[11] Harper MC. Talonavicular arthrodesis for the acquired flatfoot in the adult. Clin Orthop 1999 Aug;(365):65–8.
[12] Mann RA, Baumgarten M. Subtalar fusion for isolated subtalar disorders. Preliminary report. Clin Orthop 1988 Jan;(226):260–5.
[13] Mann RA. Talonavicular arthrodesis for the painful adult acquired flatfoot. Foot Ankle Int 1997;18(6):375–6.
[14] Mann RA, Beaman DN, Horton GA. Isolated subtalar arthrodesis. Foot Ankle Int 1998; 19(8):511–9.
[15] Mann RA, Beaman DN. Double arthrodesis in the adult. Clin Orthop 1999 Aug;(365):74–80.

[16] Toolan BC, Sangeorzan BJ, Hansen Jr ST. Complex reconstruction for the treatment of dorsolateral peritalar subluxation of the foot. Early results after distraction arthrodesis of the calcaneocuboid joint in conjunction with stabilization of, and transfer of the flexor digitorum longus tendon to, the midfoot to treat acquired pes planovalgus in adults. J Bone Joint Surg [Am] 1999;81(11):1545–60.

[17] Astion DJ, Deland JT, Otis JC, Kenneally S. Motion of the hindfoot after simulated arthrodesis. J Bone Joint Surg 1997;79:241–6.

[18] Deland JT, Otis JC, Lee KT, Kenneally SM. Lateral column lengthening with calcaneocuboid fusion: range of motion in the triple joint complex. Foot Ankle Int 1995;16(11):729–33.

[19] Gleich A. Beitzag zur operativen plattsfussbehandlung. Arch Klin Chir 1893;46:358.

[20] Koutsogiannis E. Treatment of mobile flat foot by displacement osteotomy of the calcaneus. J Bone Joint Surg [Br] 1971;53(1):96–100.

[21] Jacobs AM, Oloff LM. Surgical management of forefoot supinatus in flexible flatfoot deformity. J Foot Surg 1984;23(5):410–9.

[22] Marks RM. Medial displacement calcaneal osteotomy with flexor digitorum longus tendon substitution for stage ii posterior tibial tendon insufficiency. Tech Foot Ankle Surg 2003; 2(4):222–31.

[23] Hiller L. Surgical treatment of acquired flatfoot deformity: what is the state of practice among academic foot and ankle surgeons in 2002? Foot Ankle 2003;24(9):701–5.

[24] Laughlin TJ, Payette CR. Triple arthrodesis and subtalar joint arthrodesis. For the treatment of end-stage posterior tibial tendon dysfunction. Clin Podiatr Med Surg 1999;16(3):527–55.

[25] Cohen BE, Johnson JE. Subtalar arthrodesis for treatment of posterior tibial tendon insufficiency. Foot Ankle Clin 2001;6(1):121–8.

[26] Johnson JE, Cohen BE, DiGiovanni BF, Lamdan R. Subtalar arthrodesis with flexor digitorum longus transfer and spring ligament repair for treatment of posterior tibial tendon insufficiency. Foot Ankle Int 2000;21(9):722–9.

[27] Kitaoka HB, Patzer GL. Subtalar arthrodesis for posterior tibial tendon dysfunction and pes planus. Clin Orthop 1997;(345):187–94.

[28] Stephens HM, Walling AK, Solmen JD, Tankson CJ. Subtalar repositional arthrodesis for adult acquired flatfoot. Clin Orthop 1999 Dec;(365):69–73.

[29] Easley ME, Trnka HJ, Schon LC, Myerson MS. Isolated subtalar arthrodesis. J Bone Joint Surg [Am] 2000;82(5):613–24.

[30] McMullen S, et al. Isolated subtalar arthrodesis for posterior tibial tendon dysfunction. Paper presented at the 12th Annual Summer Meeting of the American Orthopedic Foot and Ankle Society. Hilton Head, South Carolina, 1996.

[31] Mothershed RA, Stapp MD, Smith TF. Talonavicular arthrodesis for correction of posterior tibial tendon dysfunction. Clin Podiatr Med Surg 1999;16(3):501–26.

[32] Dollard MD, Marcinko DE, Lazerson A, Elleby DH. The Evans calcaneal osteotomy for correction of flexible flatfoot syndrome. J Foot Surg 1984;23(4):291–301.

[33] Sangeorzan BJ, Mosca V, Hansen Jr ST. Effect of calcaneal lengthening on relationships among the hindfoot, midfoot, and forefoot. Foot Ankle 1993;14(3):136–41.

[34] Phillips GE. A review of elongation of os calcis for flat feet. J Bone Joint Surg [Br] 1983; 65(1):15–8.

[35] Cooper PS, Nowak MD, Shaer J. Calcaneocuboid joint pressures with lateral column lengthening (Evans) procedure. Foot Ankle Int 1997;18(4):199–205.

[36] Frankel JP, Turf RM, Kuzmicki LM. Double calcaneal osteotomy in the treatment of posterior tibial tendon dysfunction. J Foot Ankle Surg 1995;34(3):254–61.

[37] Pomeroy GC, Manoli II A. A new operative approach for flatfoot secondary to posterior tibial tendon insufficiency: a preliminary report. Foot Ankle Int 1997;18(4):206–12.

[38] Pomeroy GC, Pike RH, Beals TC, Manoli II A. Acquired flatfoot in adults due to dysfunction of the posterior tibial tendon. J Bone Joint Surg [Am] 1999;81(8):1173–82.

[39] Moseir-LaClair S, Pomeroy G, Manoli II A. Intermediate follow-up on the double osteotomy and tendon transfer procedure for stage II posterior tibial tendon insufficiency. Foot Ankle Int 2001;22(4):283–91.

[40] Mosier-LaClair S, Pomeroy G, Manoli II A. Operative treatment of the difficult stage 2 adult acquired flatfoot deformity. Foot Ankle Clin 2001;6(1):95–119.

[41] Lord JP. Correction of extreme flatfoot Value of osteotomy of os calcis and inward displacement of posterior fragment. JAMA 1923;81:1502.

[42] Silver CM, Simon SD, Spindell E, et al. Calcaneal osteotomy for valgus and varus deformities of the foot in cerebral palsy. A preliminary report on twenty-seven operations. J Bone Joint Surg [Am] 1967;49(2):232–46.

[43] Den Hartog BD. Flexor digitorum longus transfer with medial displacement calcaneal osteotomy Biomechanical rationale. Foot Ankle Clin 2001;6(1):67–76 [vi.].

[44] Catanzariti AR, Lee MS, Mendicino RW. Posterior calcaneal displacement osteotomy for adult acquired flatfoot. J Foot Ankle Surg 2000;39(1):2–14.

[45] Marks RM. Posterior tibial tendon reconstruction with medial displacement calcaneal osteotomy. Foot Ankle 1996;1:295–313.

[46] Myerson MS, Corrigan J, Thompson F, Schon LC. Tendon transfer combined with calcaneal osteotomy for treatment of posterior tibial tendon insufficiency: a radiological investigation. Foot Ankle Int 1995;16(11):712–8.

[47] Myerson MS, Corrigan J. Treatment of posterior tibial tendon dysfunction with flexor digitorum longus tendon transfer and calcaneal osteotomy. Orthopedics 1996;19(5):383–8.

[48] Weil Jr LS, Roukis TS. The calcaneal scarf osteotomy: operative technique. J Foot Ankle Surg 2001;40(3):178–82.

[49] Jacobs AM, Geistler P. Posterior calcaneal osteotomy. Effect, technique, and indications. Clin Podiatr Med Surg 1991;8(3):647–57.

[50] Jacobs AM, Oloff L, Visser HJ. Calcaneal osteotomy in the management of flexible and nonflexible flatfoot deformity: a preliminary report. J Foot Surg 1981;20(2):57–66.

[51] Jacobs AM, Sollecito V, Oloff L, Klein N. Tarsal coalitions: an instructional review. J Foot Surg 1981;20(4):214–21.

[52] Mosca VS. Calcaneal lengthening for valgus deformity of the hindfoot. Results in children who had severe, symptomatic flatfoot and skewfoot. J Bone Joint Surg [Am] 1995;77(4):500–12.

[53] Horton GA, Myerson MS, Parks BG, Park YW. Effect of calcaneal osteotomy and lateral column lengthening on the plantar fascia: a biomechanical investigation. Foot Ankle 1998;19:370–8.

[54] Thordarson DB, Hedman T, Lundquist D, Reisch R. Effect of calcaneal osteotomy and plantar fasciotomy on arch configuration in a flatfoot model. Foot Ankle Int 1998;19(6):374–8.

[55] Myerson MS, Fortin PT, Cunningham B. Changes in tibiotalar contact with calcaneal osteotomy. Trans Am Acad Orthop Surg 1994;61:149.

[56] Michelson JD, Mizel M, Jay P, Schmidt G. Effect of medial displacement calcaneal osteotomy on ankle kinematics in a cadaver model. Foot Ankle Int 1998;19(3):132–6.

[57] Steffensmeier SJ, Saltzman CL, Brown TD. Effects of medial and lateral displacement calcaneal osteotomies on tibiotalar joint contact stresses. J Orthop Res 1996;14:980–5.

[58] Guyton GP, Jeng C, Krieger LE, Mann RA. Flexor digitorum longus transfer and medial displacement calcaneal osteotomy for posterior tibial tendon dysfunction: a middle-term clinical follow-up. Foot Ankle Int 2001;22(8):627–32.

[59] Fayazi AH, Nguyen HV, Juliano PJ. Intermediate term follow-up of calcaneal osteotomy and flexor digitorum longus transfer for treatment of posterior tibial tendon dysfunction. Foot Ankle 2002;23(12):1107–11.

[60] Wacker JT, Hennessy MS, Saxby TS. Calcaneal osteotomy and transfer of the tendon flexor digitorum longus for stage-II dysfunction of tibialis posterior. Three- to five-year results. J Bone Joint Surg [Br] 2002;84(1):54–8.

ELSEVIER
SAUNDERS

Clin Podiatr Med Surg
22 (2005) 291–299

CLINICS IN
PODIATRIC
MEDICINE AND
SURGERY

Tibial Osteotomies for Lower Extremity Deformity Correction

George Vito, DPM[a],*, Floyd Pacheco, DPM[b]

[a]The Atlanta Leg Deformity Correction Center, 3556 Riverside Drive, Macon, GA 31210, USA
[b]Mercy Hospital/Barry University, 11300 NE 2nd Avenue, Miami Shores, FL 33161, USA

Lower extremity deformities and reconstruction requires a thorough understanding of the pathology and the underlining etiologies. This article reviews the basic knowledge of identifying the level of pathology and providing reconstruction of tibial deformities with osteotomies and the use of external fixation. It also provides a brief overview of proximal, midshaft, and distal tibial osteotomies and their indications.

Indications for tibial osteotomies with circular ring external fixation are numerous in the adult and pediatric patient. The more common adult indications are related to posttraumatic injury with nonunion or malunion of tibial fractures [1]. Many adults also suffer from medial column osteoarthritis of the knee with varus angular deformities of the tibia and lateral collateral ligamentous laxity. Systemic disease processes, such as rheumatoid arthritis, can influence angular deformities with resulting mechanical axis deviation and osteoarthritis in the hip, knee, and ankle joints [2].

Pediatric congenital deformities are the typical indications for corrective tibial osteotomies with circular ring external fixation. Angular deformity correction is usually required in pediatric patients with structural deformities such as tibial or fibular hemimilias and Blount's disease [2]. It is not uncommon for pediatric patients with a history of hematogionous osteomyelitis to need deformity correction as a result of growth plate arrest. Other indications include low tibial torsion and tibial varum.

---

* Corresponding author.
E-mail address: georgevito@aol.com (G. Vito).

0891-8422/05/$ – see front matter © 2005 Elsevier Inc. All rights reserved.
doi:10.1016/j.cpm.2004.12.001

The use of circular ring external fixation maximizes the optimal healing environment for patient recovery with minimal violation of soft tissue structures and vascular supply. The patient will have the advantage to be weight bearing throughout the postoperative period, minimizing the effects of disuse atrophy. Additionally, the tensioned wires provide rigid stable fixation, and with weight bearing the axial loading causes a "trampoline" effect with micromotion at the level of the osteotomy. This effect promotes a faster recovery and rapid osseous consolidation.

Clinical evaluation and preoperative management

Identifying the etiology of limb deformity is amongst the most challenging preoperative problems for the surgeon. This requires a detailed and thorough musculoskeletal examination and bilateral full-length standing radiographs [3,4]. It is extremely important identify not only the etiology of the deformity but also the level of the deformity. A combination of deformities at the hip, knee, and ankle must be examined and ruled out. Radiographs allow the clinician to evaluate the anatomical axis of each individual segment and its relationship to the mechanical axis.

The patient and family members should be given a thorough understanding on the goals and expectations of the surgery. It is important to inform the patient and parents of the use of external fixation for deformity correction, which includes proper mental preparation [2]. The family should also have an understanding of proper postoperative care, and the benefits of external fixation should be explained.

Patients and family should also be informed about the requirements that will be necessary postoperatively. This includes weekly or biweekly clinical visits as well as daily appointments with physical therapy. This is dependent on the deformity correction, and patients are encouraged to be weight bearing during the postoperative period to tolerance.

Mechanical axis in relation to uniapical and multiapical deformities

Assessment of the deformity is typically identified with the use of bilateral full-length weight-bearing radiographs. The mechanical and anatomical axes are identified and described based on normal values as described by Paley and Testworth [5,6]. Deformity is identified based on deviation of magnitude, plane, and direction from the normal mechanical axis. The apex of a deformity is located based on the radiographic mechanical axis of each segment of the deformity. The bisection of the mechanical axis of each segment identifies the center of rotation of angulation (CORA) and the degree of the deformity. Multisegmental involvement requires evaluation of each individual deformity and its mechanical axis relation [5,6].

The mechanical axis is defined as the static weight-bearing axis. In the frontal plane it is identified with a line drawn on radiographs from the center of the femoral head to the center of the ankle joint [5,6]. Normal mechanical axis in the frontal plane passes slightly medial to the center of the tibial spine of the knee joint. Lateral weight-bearing radiographs are required to identify the mechanical axis in the sagittal plane. This is identified with a line that is anterior to S2 and extends inferiorly and slightly posterior to the center of the femoral head and extends inferiorly to the center of the ankle joint. Normally the line should be in alignment with the center of gravity that is located slightly anterior to the knee joint. Deviation and deformity of the mechanical axis is identified and measured in millimeters.

Angular deformities can be situated in any plane, and it is important to identify the multiplanar deformities and understand their malalignment relationship to the mechanical axis. The oblique axis of the deformity can be calculated based on frontal and sagittal plane radiographic measurements. This may also involve a combinational translation deformity [5,6].

Once the deformity and segmental involvement has been identified, the mechanical axis of each segment of the deformity must be evaluated according to the nonpathological contralateral limb or through trigonometric measurements obtained from the frontal plane and sagittal plane radiographs. These measurements are identified based on the tangent of the proximal or distal segment of the deformity to the nonpathological hip, knee, or ankle joint respectively [5,6].

Fixation blocks and working length

It is necessary to explain the basic vocabulary and concepts that are involved with the anticipated apparatus design for angular correction of the tibia. Fixation of corticotomies that are juxtaarticular at the proximal or distal tibia typically require a single-ring tibial fixation block adjacent to the joint. It is ideal to have two rings of fixation per segment of bone, but because of the intimate location of the osteotomy in relation to the joint a single ring is required.

Two-ring tibial fixation blocks are assembled with the connection of two individual rings with four threaded rods. This portion of the apparatus is used to control a longer segment of bone and is typically part of the apparatus design for three-ring constructs that are used for proximal and distal tibial angular correction and corticotomies.

A five-eighths ring with a supporting ring is another form of fixation block that is typically used at the proximal tibial region when tibial osteotomy is performed for limb-length discrepancy and monofocal bone transport. The block is arranged with the five-eighths ring as the superior ring and it is connected to a full ring with 3- to 4-cm sockets [7]. This provides strength to the open five-eighths ring. Tensioned wires on this open ring would result in deformation of the ring, and the supporting ring below is necessary to prevent this. The open portion of the five-eighths ring is positioned posteriorly to allow for active and passive range of motion of the knee joint without soft tissue impingement [7].

Working-length rings are defined as a single ring that is typically used in bone transport. It travels along the working length at a rate of 1 mm per day for osseous and soft tissue generation. The working length is defined as the distance between two fixation blocks [7].

Tibial osteotomies

Varus and valgus angular deformity correction at any level of the tibia requires that the proximal segment of the pathological tibia be bisected at the mechanical axis or perpendicular to the adjacent joint. The distal portion of the tibial deformity is also bisected at the mechanical axis [5–9]. The bisection of these lines is identified as the level of the deformity. It is at this level that hinges must be placed at 90 degrees to the plane of the deformity, and push rods should be spaced symmetrically in the same plane to provide distraction and angular correction.

If the degree of angular deformity is high, these push rods may require hinge placement to accommodate the position of the concave portion of the deformity.

Proximal tibial osteotomies

Genu varum and genu valgum require a minimum of three rings for angular correction. The normal anatomical and mechanical axes form an identical single line that is slightly medial to the tibial spine. The level of the deformity is identified and preparation for the corticotomy is performed.

An approximately 2-cm incision is placed at the distal one third of the lateral aspect of the fibula. Dissection is carried down to identify the fibula, and using an osteotome or sagital saw, a fibular corticotomy is performed. This can be either transverse or oblique. The area is irrigated and deep tissues are reapproximated with absorbable sutures. The epidermis is reapproximated with skin staples.

Fluoroscopy is used to identify the knee joint, level of the anticipated placement of the proximal single ring fixation block, and the level of the anticipated corticotomy. A skin scribe is used to mark each of these levels on the leg.

Two small incisions approximately 1.5 cm in length are performed over the anticipated corticotomy at the level of the angular deformity. One incision is placed along the central anterior-medial face, and the second incision is placed lateral to the anterior tibial crest. Both incisions are performed in a longitudinal orientation. The periosteum is minimally incised and reflected using an elevator.

Two large right-angle forceps are required for percutaneous placement of a gigli saw to encompass the tibia for proximal tibial corticotomy. Umbilical tape is used to thread the gigli saw around the tibia at the level of the proximal metaphysis. The umbilical tape is looped onto itself to form an anchoring device for the right-angle forceps. The right-angle forceps are inserted subperiostally through both incisions. The umbilical tape is entered from medial and threaded posterior to the tibia to the adjacent right-angle forcep through the lateral incision. The umbilical tape is pulled through the lateral incision. The gigli saw is anchored to the umbilical tape and then passed through the incisions to encompass the tibia subperiosteally.

The gigli saw is secured to the anterior soft tissues temporarily while the external fixation apparatus is applied. The tibial corticotomy should not be performed until the external fixation apparatus is applied and all wires are tensioned. It is easier to fixate a stable bone segment and this prevents enhancing angular deformity with placement of wires into an unstable distal segment.

Corticotomy can also be performed with the use of an osteotome and mallet. This would be performed through a single incision approximately 2 cm in length on the medial face of the tibia, at the end of the procedure after the fixation has been applied. The working length rods are removed temporarily to allow for external rotation of the distal segment to complete the corticotomy of the posterior lateral cortex.

The circular ring external fixation device is applied next. Proximal tibial angular correction is performed acutely or gradually depending on the degree of angulation. Deformities with higher degrees of angulation require gradual correction. Postoperative complications should be anticipated and it is best to use four hinges for the working length between the single-ring tibial fixation block and the two-ring distal tibial fixation block.

The active hinges should be placed 90 degrees to the plane of the deformity. Varus and valgus deformities of the knee will have hinges situated at the convex portion of the deformity [5–9]. One hinge is placed anterior and the other is placed posterior. These are placed at varying degrees based on the deformity, and proper placement is important to prevent translation and impingement of the convex cortex. Opening osteotomies with bone grafting are not necessary, and closing wedge osteotomies are not performed because of limb shortening. Varus angular correction is eliminated with placement of hinges 90 degrees to the plane of the apex of the deformity, and gradual lengthening of push rods at the concave side of the deformity is performed at a rate of 1 mm per day.

The single-ring fixation block is applied to the proximal portion of the knee perpendicular to the anatomical bisection of the proximal tibia and perpendicular to the anatomical axis. Fixation should be 1 to 2 cm below the identified knee joint to prevent inadvertent penetration of the joint capsule or placement of intraarticular wires. A horizontal lateral to medial olive reference wire is placed and is secured to the ring with slotted bolts and nuts.

Orthogonal placement of the rings is evaluated to allow 2 to 3 cm of soft tissue clearance circumferentially. A second reference wire is placed at the level of the distal tibial ring of the two-ring distal tibial fixation block. This ring is secured approximately 5 cm proximal to the ankle joint. The reference wire is placed from medial to lateral with an olive wire. The wire is secured to the ring with slotted bolts and nuts.

Orthogonal placement is again evaluated, and if the position is satisfactory then the frame is "locked" into position. If unsatisfactory, the frame can be modified medial to lateral with light tapping of the frame with a mallet to the desired position. Anterior to posterior placement can be modified with repositioning of the slotted bolts on the ring. If the surgeon is not satisfied and the wires are not properly placed, the wires should be removed and redirected to the desired position. If the surgeon continues to place wires with unsatisfactory position, the frame cannot be modified once it is locked. All wires would need to be removed and redirected.

Once satisfactory position is achieved, the frame is locked. A second olive wire is placed from posterior medial to anterior lateral with special care to avoid the posterior medial gastrocnemius and pes anserinus structures and the patellar tendon anteriorly. This would be irritating to the patient and prevent range of motion at the knee joint.

A third wire is placed through the head of the fibula and directed anterior-medially. An angle of 60 degrees is formed with proper placement of these two wires as they exit the bone medially and laterally [7].

The distal ring of the two-ring distal tibial fixation block is locked with an olive wire from posterior lateral to anterior medial. A third wire is directed from posterior medial to anterior lateral. The frame is considered to be locked, and the position is committed.

All wires on the proximal tibial single-ring fixation block and the distal tibial ring of the two-ring tibial fixation block are secured and tensioned in the proper manner. Attention is directed toward securing the proximal ring of the distal tibial two-ring fixation block. This is done with a medial to lateral wire and a medial face wire from posterior medial to anterior lateral. Wires are secured and tensioned in the proper fashion.

Two final and important wires are placed. The first wire is placed inferior to the proximal single-ring fixation block approximately 3 cm proximal to the anticipated area of tibial corticotomy. This is placed from medial to lateral, and three- or four-hole posts are used to secure this wire. The second wire is placed superior to the proximal ring of the two-ring distal tibial fixation block and approximately 3 cm distal to the anticipated corticotomy site. Both wires are secured and tensioned between 70 to 90 kg. These two wires control the leaver arm of each bone segment and assist in preventing malalignment and drifting at the corticotomy site.

Proper hinge placement is evaluated to ensure that they are placed at the apex of the deformity along the convex aspect. The hinges should be approximately 90 degrees to the plane of the deformity (see references [4–7,9]). The gigli saw corticotomy is finally performed and the incision sites are reapproximated with nonabsorbable suture. Angular correction is corrected gradually at a rate of 1 mm per day with distraction of the opposing push rods.

Midshaft tibial osteotomies

The same hinge concepts and principles apply to midshaft osteotomies. The only difference is within the design of the apparatus. A midshaft tibial diaphyseal deformity allows for two-ring proximal and distal tibial fixation blocks to be applied above and below the anticipated corticotomy site. This provides a stable and rigid construct of the longer leaver arms of both segments.

The working length is that distance between the proximal and distal two-ring tibial fixation blocks. Hinges are placed at the appropriate 90 degrees to the plane of the deformity, and if the amount of angular correction is severe the push rods should be extended off the ring with extended plates.

Rigidity can be improved with replacement of hinged rods with straight threaded rods after gradual correction has taken place and proper alignment is achieved. The threaded rods will be shortened to provide compression.

Distal tibial osteotomies

Correction of distal tibial angular deformities is similar to techniques used for proximal tibial osteotomies. A three-ring apparatus design is used and the apex of the deformity is identified in the usual manner. Corticotomy is performed at the appropriate level with hinges approximately 90 degrees to the apex of the deformity.

If instability is sufficient as a result of osteotomy of the tibia and fibula at the distal aspect, then the ankle joint can be spanned with a foot plate or a half-ring. This will enhance rigidity of the frame and the foot plate or half-ring may be removed once angular correction has been achieved gradually and held in position for 3 to 4 weeks.

The use of tibial osteotomy to restore alignment of the ankle joint mechanical axis has proven beneficial in studies by Myerson [10,11]. Patients who suffer from osteoarthritis of the ankle were reported to have less pain and improved function with or without radiographic improvement. The major complications of distal tibial corticotomies include translational deformities, delayed union, and nonunion [2,10–16]. It is best to perform such osteotomies with circular ring external fixation rather than internal fixation to allow for proper post-operative correction and manipulation as well as allow the patient to be weight bearing.

Summary

Lower extremity deformity correction with transosseous osteosynthesis and angular correction are common in pediatric patients and posttraumatic events in the adult. It is important that the surgeon identifies the level of the deformity and deviation of the mechanical axis. Radiographic angles and trigonometric calculations identify triplanar deformities and the center of rotation of angulation. These are the minimum requirements to identifying the involved pathological segments of the lower extremity deformity.

Proper identification of the level of deformity allows the surgeon to apply hinges within the pathological plane of the deformity. This is defined as the plane 90 degrees to the apex of deformity or the center of rotation of angulation. The understanding of circular ring external fixation biomechanics and mechanization are also required for the desired successful outcome. This article provided a general overview of identification of tibial deformities and the deviation from the normal mechanical axis of the lower extremity.

It is important that the surgeon understands that each lower-extremity pathology is unique and requires a focused and individual work-up. Apparatus designs are never identical, and the designs described are based on the basic biomechanics of circular ring external fixation and the role that it plays in deformity correction of the tibia and restoration of the anatomical and mechanical axis.

References

[1] McMaster M. Disability of the hindfoot after fracture of the tibial shaft. J Bone Joint Surg [Br] 1976;58(1):90–3.
[2] Heywood AW. Supramalleolar osteotomy in the management of the rheumatoid hindfoot. Clin Orthop 1983;4:76–81.
[3] Chao EY, Neluheni EV, Hsu RW, Paley E. Biomechanics of malalignment. Orthop Clin North Am 1994;25:379–86.
[4] Dahl M, Gulli B, Berg T. Complications of limb lengthening. A learning curve. Clin Orthop 1994;1(201):10–8.
[5] Paley D, Testworth K. Mechanical axis deviation of the lower limbs; preoperative planning of multiapical frontal plane angular deformities of the femur and tibia. Clin Orthop 1992; 3(280):65–71.
[6] Paley D, Testworth K. Mechanical axis deviaton of the lower limbs: preoperative planning of uniapical angular deformities of the tibia and femur. Clin Orthop 1992;6(280):48–64.
[7] Hutson J. Basic frame construction: building fixation blocks and designing working length mechanization. Tech Orthop 2002;17(1):26–33.
[8] Catagni MA, Kirienko VMA. Tibial angular deformities. Advances in Ilizarov apparatus assembly. Lippincott Williams & Wilkins; 1994. p. 101–12.
[9] Paley D, Testworth K. Mal-alignment and realignment of the lower extremity. Orthop Clin North Am 1994;25:367–77.
[10] Hall RL. The use of osteotomy to correct foot and ankle deformities. In: Myerson MS, editor. Foot and ankle disorders. Philadelphia: WB Saunders; 2000. p. 94–9.
[11] Mangone PG. Distal tibial osteotomies for the treatment of foot and ankle disorders. Foot Ankle Clin 2001;6:583–97.

[12] McNicol D, Leong JCY, Hsu LCS. Supramalleolar derotation osteotomy for lateral tibial torsion and associated equinovarus deformity of the foot. J Bone Joint Surg [Br] 1983;65(2):166–70.

[13] Abraham E, Lubicky J, Songer MN, Millar EA. Supramalleolar osteotomy for ankle valgus in myelomeningocele. J Pediatr Orthop 1996;16:774–81.

[14] Acevedo J, Myerson M. Reconstruction alternatives for ankle arthritis. Foot Ankle Clin 1999; 11:409–30.

[15] Graehl P, Hersh M, et al. Supramalleolar osteotomy for the treatment of symptomatic tibial malunion. J Othrop Trauma 1998;1:281–92.

[16] Waanders NA, Herzenberg JE. The theoretical application of inclinded hinges with the Ilizarov external fixator for simultaneous angulation and rotation correction. Bull Hosp Joint Dis 1992; 52(1):27–32.

ELSEVIER
SAUNDERS

Clin Podiatr Med Surg
22 (2005) 301–307

CLINICS IN
PODIATRIC
MEDICINE AND
SURGERY

Long Arm Decompression Osteotomy for Hallux Limitus

Stephen C. Robinson, DPM[a],*, Ryan P. Frank, DPM[b]

[a]4240 Blue Ridge Boulevard, Raytown, MO 64133, USA
[b]2406 East R.D. Mize Road, Independence, MO 64057, USA

Hallux limitus/rigidus is a progressive degeneration of the first metatarsophalangeal joint. When left untreated, this joint may advance through increasingly severe stages of arthrosis as described by Regnauld [1], and later modified by Drago et al [2]. When a patient presents with stage I or II hallux limitus, a joint preservation surgical procedure may be indicated. As the degeneration of the first metatarsophalangeal joint becomes more severe, joint destructive procedures become the treatment of choice when considering surgical options. This article introduces a new distal first metatarsal osteotomy, which may be used for treatment of stage I or II hallux limitus.

Indications

The long arm decompression osteotomy (LADO) of the first metatarsal is indicated for a specific group of patients with hallux limitus. Patients should be classified as having stage I or II hallux limitus and be good candidates for a joint preservation procedure. This osteotomy is indicated in patients with mild to moderate metatarsus primus elevatus or an abnormally long first metatarsal. The LADO can be used to shorten the first metatarsal or plantarflex the first metatarsal head.

---

* Corresponding author.

0891-8422/05/$ – see front matter © 2005 Elsevier Inc. All rights reserved.
doi:10.1016/j.cpm.2004.11.003
podiatric.theclinics.com

Surgical technique

A standard dorsomedial linear longitudinal incision is made over the first metatarsophalangeal joint. Following dissection of the subcutaneous tissues, a linear longitudinal capsulotomy is performed over the dorsal first metatarsophalangeal joint. The capsular structures are then reflected medially and laterally, exposing the first metatarsal head. At this point, a cheilectomy is performed to remove any osteophytes that may be restricting motion [3]. Additionally, the joint surfaces at the head of the first metatarsal and the base of the first proximal phalanx are examined, and, if necessary, a fenestration chondroplasty is performed to promote fibrocartilage growth at articular surface defects [4].

The amount of plantarflexion and shortening of the first metatarsal is determined preoperatively. Comparison of the length of the first and second rays should be made with radiographs, with the postsurgical goal of achieving equal lengths or shorter first ray by 1 to 2 mm. A V-type osteotomy is performed in the metaphyseal region of the first metatarsal. The osteotomy is made dorsally to plantarly, with the apex pointing distally, and a longer medial arm to accommodate internal fixation. The proximal aspect of the medial arm should exit somewhere in the middle third of the first metatarsal. The osteotomy is similar to a V-type dorsal to plantar osteotomy that can be made to elevate a lesser metatarsal, with the exception of the longer medial arm. When performing this osteotomy, it is important to angle the saw blade slightly from dorsal distal to plantar proximal at the apex to avoid the sesamoid apparatus. An axis guide may be used if the surgeon wishes. If more than 1 to 2 mm of shortening of the first metatarsal is desired, a second osteotomy is performed on the first metatarsal shaft (Fig. 1). This second osteotomy should be made on both arms,

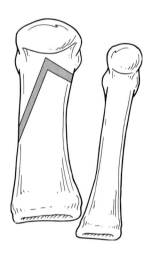

Fig. 1. Schematic demonstrating dorsal to plantar LADO with a second osteotomy proximal and parallel to the first osteotomy. The section of bone between osteotomies is then removed.

equal and parallel to the first osteotomy. The section of bone is then removed. It is important to remove sections from both the medial and lateral arms for two reasons. First, this will achieve accurate, predictable shortening and second, removing a section from both arms prevents medial or lateral translation of the capital fragment. When determining the width of this section of bone to be removed one should expect that the first osteotomy will produce 1 to 2 mm of shortening because of the width of the blade. In the authors' opinion, this second osteotomy represents the most technically challenging aspect of the procedure because of the difficulty of maintaining an osteotomy parallel to the first osteotomy.

The capital fragment is then transposed plantarly and impacted on the first metatarsal shaft. Fixation is achieved through one or two screws driven from distal medial to proximal lateral across the medial arm of the capital fragment. The author has found one 2.7-mm cortical bone screw to be sufficient. Following fixation, the bony prominence at the dorsal aspect of the osteotomy and the proximal aspect of the medial arm are resected. Correction of the deformity is then assessed visually and with intraoperative radioagraphy. Range of motion is checked with the foot loaded and unloaded. The incision is flushed and closed in layers.

Postoperative care

A sterile compressive dressing is applied and the patient is instructed to remain non–weight bearing for the first 2 weeks postoperatively. A posterior splint may be used if so desired. A dressing change is performed at 1 week postoperatively, followed by suture removal at week 2. After 2 weeks the patient is allowed to bear weight in a rigid surgical shoe but advised to limit ambulation. The patient is also instructed to perform first metatarsophalangeal joint range-of-motion exercises at week 2 postoperatively. If there is clinical and radiographic evidence of osseous union at week 6, the patient is allowed to return to normal shoe gear and advised to continue range-of-motion exercises. The patient may be discharged if doing well at 10 weeks postoperatively.

Advantages/disadvantages of LADO versus other joint-preserving procedures

The LADO will allow approximately 4 to 6 mm of plantarflexion of the first metatarsal (Fig. 2). This range should fall somewhere between the amount of plantarflexion achieved with a distal osteotomy versus a proximal osteotomy. For severe elevatus, a more proximal osteotomy would be the procedure of choice as the LADO would not achieve enough plantarflexion. However, when a lesser amount of plantarflexion is needed, the LADO provides some specific advantages. With the LADO it is much easier to visualize the amount of

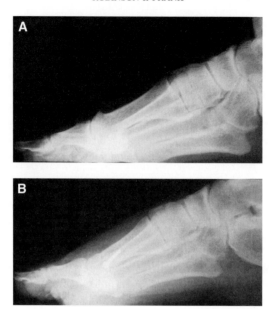

Fig. 2. (*A*) Preoperative weight-bearing lateral radiograph showing moderate metatarsus primus elevatus. (*B*) Postoperative weight bearing lateral radiograph showing plantarflexion achieved of first metatarsal.

plantarflexion that has been achieved. Because the LADO is a dorsal-to-plantar osteotomy and the capital fragment is transposed directly plantarly, the amount of plantarflexion is more predictable and controllable. With the Youngswick modification of the Austin osteotomy, it has been shown that the amount of plantarflexion is dependent on the angle of the plantar cut, in addition to the section of bone resected dorsally [5].

The LADO is easy to fixate. However, it is important to ensure that the capital fragment is impacted upon the metatarsal shaft to avoid rotation of the metatarsal head. Any dorsal rotation at the osteotomy site would negate the effect of the plantarflexion of the distal fragment. Because the medial arm is made longer, it accommodates one or two screws from medial to lateral across this arm. If a single screw is used it is recommended that it be driven at an angle halfway between perpendicular to the osteotomy and perpendicular to the long axis of the metatarsal.

The LADO is believed to be more stable than a proximal osteotomy and less stable than a typical distal osteotomy. Because of the placement of the osteotomy in the metaphyseal region, there would be a shorter lever arm at this point compared with a more proximal osteotomy, thus providing less stress at the osteotomy. The LADO is oriented dorsally to plantarly; therefore, it is believed to be less stable than a typical distal first metatarsal osteotomy. This is why patients are kept non–weight bearing for the first 2 weeks following a LADO. Additionally, as mentioned previously the cuts are angle from dorsal distal to proximal plantar to avoid the sesamoid apparatus. This angulation of the cuts also provides some additional stability to this procedure.

The LADO avoids periosteal stripping of the entire first metatarsal. With most joint-preserving procedures it is desirable to perform a cheilectomy and also possibly a chrondroplasty. If the surgeon chooses to perform a proximal first metatarsal osteotomy in conjunction with cheilectomy or chondroplasty, it becomes necessary to perform extensive dissection and virtually deglove the entire first metatarsal. When a LADO is performed, a standard dorsal first metatarsophalangeal joint capsulotomy is performed and the joint is exposed.

Troughing may be less likely with the LADO as compared with the dorsal to plantar Z-type osteotomy for hallux limitus. It is well documented that troughing may occur with the scarf-type osteotomy for hallux valgus [6]. The same complication may also occur with the dorsal to plantar Z-type osteotomy for hallux limitus. There is more bone-to-bone interface with the LADO because the osteotomy is in the metaphyseal region of the bone. Troughing may occur with the LADO if the distal fragment is plantarflexed too aggressively.

The LADO may be used to correct an excessively long first metatarsal (Fig. 3). Virtually any amount of shortening can be achieved with this procedure. The authors estimate that the first osteotomy will shorten the metatarsal by 1 to 2 mm because of the width of the saw blade. It is vital to accurately estimate the amount of shortening desired preoperatively and to take into account the width of the blade when making calculations. It is recommended that the metatarsal protrusion distance be measured on AP radiographs [7]. For

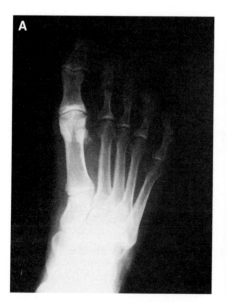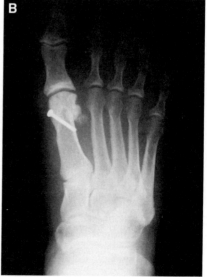

Fig. 3. (*A*) Preoperative weight-bearing AP radiograph showing elongated first metatarsal. (*B*) Postoperative weight-bearing AP radiograph showing shortening achieved of first metatarsal.

example, if 5 mm of shortening of the first metatarsal is desired, the section of bone removed from the metatarsal should measure approximately 2 mm. This is estimating that the first metatarsal will be shortened by 2 to 4 mm from the two osteotomies alone in addition to the width of bone resected. If 2 to 3 mm of shortening is the goal, then two blades of the same size may be placed on the saw adjacent to each other, and a single wider cut is made.

There is some risk that the cut at the apex may interfere with the sesamoid apparatus. It is important to angle the saw blade from dorsal distal to plantar proximal at this point. An axis guide may also be used to ensure proper angulation of this cut. If the apical cut did encounter the sesamoids it could potentially lead to arthritis at the first metatarsal sesamoid articulation. Either a sagittal saw or an oscillating saw may be used to make the osteotomy cuts. The second osteotomy seems to be the most technically challenging aspect of the procedure. It is important to make the second cuts parallel to the first to ensure good bone-to-bone contact at all points along the osteotomy.

The LADO as described does not allow any correction of first and second intermetatarsal angle deformity and should not be considered in cases of hallux limitus with increased first intermetatarsal angle. This procedure will not allow for correction in the transverse or frontal planes. The correction achieved with the LADO will be in the form of shortening the metatarsal and sagittal plane correction.

Summary

The LADO represents a new approach to stage I and II hallux limitus. It is possible to achieve more correction in length and in the sagittal plane with this osteotomy as compared with other distal first metatarsal osteotomies. The LADO may be more stable than proximal osteotomies. The senior author has recently begun using the LADO for selected patients. So far, only two procedures have been performed, with excellent results on both patients. The LADO has not replaced other distal osteotomies but instead has become another option in patients who need up to 5 mm of plantarflexion or some degree of shortening of the first metatarsal.

References

[1] Regnauld B. Hallux rigidus. In: Regnauld B, editor. The foot. Berlin: Springer-Verlag; 1986. p. 345–59.
[2] Drago JJ, Oloff L, Jacobs AM. A comprehensive review of hallux limitus. J Foot Surg 1984; 23(3):213–20.
[3] Geldwert JJ, Rock GD, McGrath MP, Mancusso JE. Cheilectomy: still a useful technique for grade I and grade II hallux limitus/rigidus. J Foot Surg 1992;31(2):154–9.
[4] Kissel CG, Nagaria J, Stephens M. Cheilectomy, chondroplasty, and sagittal "Z" osteotomy:

a preliminary report on an alternative joint preservation approach to hallux limitus. J Foot Ankle Surg 1995;34(3):312–8.

[5] Gerbert J, Moadab A, Rupley KF. Youngswick-Austin procedure: the effect of plantar arm orientation on metatarsal head displacement. J Foot Ankle Surg 2001;40(1):8–14.

[6] Coetzee JC. Scarf osteotomy for hallux valgus repair: the dark side. Foot Ankle Int 2003; 24(1):29–33.

[7] Palladino SJ. Preoperative evaluation of the bunion patient: etiology, biomechanics, clinical and radiographic assessment. In: Gerbert J, editor. Textbook of bunion surgery. Mt. Kisco (NY): Futura; 1991. p. 1–88.

ELSEVIER
SAUNDERS

Clin Podiatr Med Surg
22 (2005) 309–314

CLINICS IN
PODIATRIC
MEDICINE AND
SURGERY

Index

Note: Page numbers of article titles are in **boldface** type.

A

Abductor digiti minimi muscle, myectomy of, for tailor's bunionette, 243

Achilles tendon, lengthening of, with posterior calcaneal displacement osteotomy, 279

Akinette osteotomy, of proximal phalanx, with central metatarsal osteotomy, 219

Allen modification, of Wilson osteotomy, for hallux valgus, 146

Ankle joint, deformities of, tibial osteotomy for, 297

Arthrodesis
calcaneocuboid joint distraction, for posterior tibial tendon dysfunction, 285
proximal interphalangeal joint, with central metatarsal osteotomy, 213, 215
talonavicular, for posterior tibial tendon dysfunction, 285
tarsometatarsal, for cavus foot, 255
triple, for cavus foot, 256

Austin osteotomy, for hallux valgus, 149–155

Avascular necrosis, from distal metatarsal osteotomy, for hallux valgus, 162–165

B

Barouk-Rippstein-Toulec osteotomy, of metatarsal, for tailor's bunionette, 242

Bicorrectional chevron osteotomy, for hallux valgus, 154–155

Biplane, double step-off osteotomy (Mitchell), for hallux valgus, 145–146

Block test, in cavus foot, 249

Bone graft, in Evans calcaneal osteotomy, 271–273

B.R.T. (Barouk-Rippstein-Toulec) osteotomy, of metatarsal, for tailor's bunionette, 242

Bunion. *See* Hallux valgus.

Bunionectomy
midshaft osteotomies in. *See* Hallux valgus, midshaft osteotomies for.
simple, for tailor's bunionette, 225–229

Bunionette, tailor's. *See* Tailor's bunionette.

C

Calcaneocuboid joint
arthrosis of, Evans procedure contraindications in, 266
distraction arthrodesis of, for posterior tibial tendon dysfunction, 285

Calcaneometatarsal angle, in cavus foot, 249

Calcaneus, osteotomy of
Evans. *See* Evans calcaneal osteotomy.
for cavus foot, 255, 260
posterior. *See* Posterior calcaneal displacement osteotomy.

Callus, in cavus foot, 248

Cavus foot, **247–264**
classification of, 250
conditions associated with, 250–252
conservative treatment of, 252
definition of, 247–248
etiology of, 247–248
evaluation of, 248–250
surgical treatment of, 252–262
calcaneal osteotomy in, 255–256
Jahss procedure for, 255
Lapidus procedure in, 254
midfoot osteotomies in, 256–262
soft tissue procedures in, 253
tendon transfers in, 253–254

Central metatarsal(s), **197–222**
disorders of
causes of, 197–198
conservative treatment of, 198
osteotomies of, 200
concomitant lesser digit procedures with, 213–219

doi:10.1016/S0891-8422(05)00024-8

podiatric.theclinics.com

Changing Your Address?

Make sure your subscription changes too! When you notify us of your new address, you can help make our job easier by including an exact copy of your Clinics label number with your old address (see illustration below.) This number identifies you to our computer system and will speed the processing of your address change. Please be sure this label number accompanies your old address and your corrected address—you can send an old Clinics label with your number on it or just copy it exactly and send it to the address listed below.

We appreciate your help in our attempt to give you continuous coverage. Thank you.

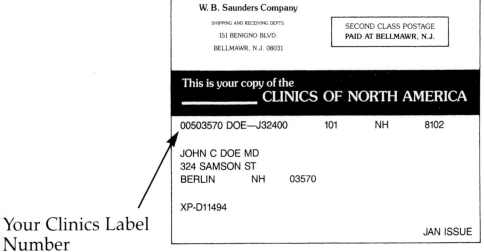

W. B. Saunders Company

SHIPPING AND RECEIVING DEPTS.

151 BENIGNO BLVD.

BELLMAWR, N.J. 08031

SECOND CLASS POSTAGE
PAID AT BELLMAWR, N.J.

This is your copy of the
_____ **CLINICS OF NORTH AMERICA**

00503570 DOE—J32400   101   NH   8102

JOHN C DOE MD
324 SAMSON ST
BERLIN   NH   03570

XP-D11494

JAN ISSUE

Your Clinics Label Number

Copy it exactly or send your label
along with your address to:
W.B. Saunders Company, Customer Service
Orlando, FL 32887-4800
Call Toll Free 1-800-654-2452

Please allow four to six weeks for delivery of new subscriptions and for processing address changes.

Order your subscription today. Simply complete and detach this card and drop it in the mail to receive the best clinical information in your field.

❑ **Adolescent Medicine Clinics**
- ❑ Individual $95
- ❑ Institutions $133
- ❑ *In-training $48

❑ **Anesthesiology**
- ❑ Individual $175
- ❑ Institutions $270
- ❑ *In-training $88

❑ **Cardiology**
- ❑ Individual $170
- ❑ Institutions $266
- ❑ *In-training $85

❑ **Chest Medicine**
- ❑ Individual $185
- ❑ Institutions $285

❑ **Child and Adolescent Psychiatry**
- ❑ Individual $175
- ❑ Institutions $265
- ❑ *In-training $88

❑ **Critical Care**
- ❑ Individual $165
- ❑ Institutions $266
- ❑ *In-training $83

❑ **Dental**
- ❑ Individual $150
- ❑ Institutions $242

❑ **Emergency Medicine**
- ❑ Individual $170
- ❑ Institutions $263
- ❑ *In-training $85
  - ❑ Send CME info

❑ **Facial Plastic Surgery**
- ❑ Individual $199
- ❑ Institutions $300

❑ **Foot and Ankle**
- Individual $160
- Institutions $232

❑ **Gastroenterology**
- ❑ Individual $190
- ❑ Institutions $276

❑ **Gastrointestinal Endoscopy**
- ❑ Individual $190
- ❑ Institutions $276

❑ **Hand**
- ❑ Individual $205
- ❑ Institutions $319

❑ **Heart Failure (NEW in 2005!)**
- ❑ Individual $99
- ❑ Institutions $149
- ❑ *In-training $49

❑ **Hematology/ Oncology**
- ❑ Individual $210
- ❑ Institutions $315

❑ **Immunology & Allergy**
- ❑ Individual $165
- ❑ Institutions $266

❑ **Infectious Disease**
- ❑ Individual $165
- ❑ Institutions $272

❑ **Clinics in Liver Disease**
- ❑ Individual $165
- ❑ Institutions $234

❑ **Medical**
- ❑ Individual $140
- ❑ Institutions $244
- ❑ *In-training $70
  - ❑ Send CME info

❑ **MRI**
- ❑ Individual $190
- ❑ Institutions $290
- ❑ *In-training $95
  - ❑ Send CME info

❑ **Neuroimaging**
- ❑ Individual $190
- ❑ Institutions $290
- ❑ *In-training $95
  - ❑ Send CME info

❑ **Neurologic**
- ❑ Individual $175
- ❑ Institutions $275

❑ **Obstetrics & Gynecology**
- ❑ Individual $175
- ❑ Institutions $288

❑ **Occupational and Environmental Medicine**
- ❑ Individual $120
- ❑ Institutions $166
- ❑ *In-training $60

❑ **Ophthalmology**
- ❑ Individual $190
- ❑ Institutions $325

❑ **Oral & Maxillofacial Surgery**
- ❑ Individual $180
- ❑ Institutions $280
- ❑ *In-training $90

❑ **Orthopedic**
- ❑ Individual $180
- ❑ Institutions $295
- ❑ *In-training $90

❑ **Otolaryngologic**
- ❑ Individual $199
- ❑ Institutions $350

❑ **Pediatric**
- ❑ Individual $135
- ❑ Institutions $246
- ❑ *In-training $68
  - ❑ Send CME info

❑ **Perinatology**
- ❑ Individual $155
- ❑ Institutions $237
- ❑ *In-training $78
  - ❑ Send CME inf0

❑ **Plastic Surgery**
- ❑ Individual $245
- ❑ Institutions $370

❑ **Podiatric Medicine & Surgery**
- ❑ Individual $170
- ❑ Institutions $266

❑ **Primary Care**
- ❑ Individual $135
- ❑ Institutions $223

❑ **Psychiatric**
- ❑ Individual $170
- ❑ Institutions $288

❑ **Radiologic**
- ❑ Individual $220
- ❑ Institutions $331
- ❑ *In-training $110
  - ❑ Send CME info

❑ **Sports Medicine**
- ❑ Individual $180
- ❑ Institutions $277

❑ **Surgical**
- ❑ Individual $190
- ❑ Institutions $299
- ❑ *In-training $95

❑ **Thoracic Surgery (formerly Chest Surgery)**
- ❑ Individual $175
- ❑ Institutions $255
- ❑ *In-training $88

❑ **Urologic**
- ❑ Individual $195
- ❑ Institutions $307
- ❑ *In-training $98
  - ❑ Send CME info

BUSINESS REPLY MAIL

FIRST-CLASS MAIL   PERMIT NO 7135   ORLANDO FL

POSTAGE WILL BE PAID BY ADDRESSEE

PERIODICALS ORDER FULFILLMENT DEPT
ELSEVIER
6277 SEA HARBOR DR
ORLANDO FL 32821-9816